THE COMPLETE
RUNNER'S
DAY-BY-DAY LOG
2021 CALENDAR

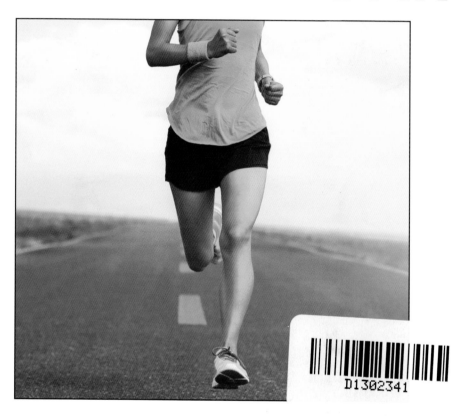

D1302341

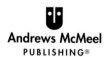

Andrews McMeel
PUBLISHING®

MARTY JEROME

2020

January
S	M	T	W	T	F	S
			1	2	3	4
5	6	7	8	9	10	11
12	13	14	15	16	17	18
19	20	21	22	23	24	25
26	27	28	29	30	31	

February
S	M	T	W	T	F	S
						1
2	3	4	5	6	7	8
9	10	11	12	13	14	15
16	17	18	19	20	21	22
23	24	25	26	27	28	29

March
S	M	T	W	T	F	S
1	2	3	4	5	6	7
8	9	10	11	12	13	14
15	16	17	18	19	20	21
22	23	24	25	26	27	28
29	30	31				

April
S	M	T	W	T	F	S
			1	2	3	4
5	6	7	8	9	10	11
12	13	14	15	16	17	18
19	20	21	22	23	24	25
26	27	28	29	30		

May
S	M	T	W	T	F	S
					1	2
3	4	5	6	7	8	9
10	11	12	13	14	15	16
17	18	19	20	21	22	23
24	25	26	27	28	29	30
31						

June
S	M	T	W	T	F	S
	1	2	3	4	5	6
7	8	9	10	11	12	13
14	15	16	17	18	19	20
21	22	23	24	25	26	27
28	29	30				

July
S	M	T	W	T	F	S
			1	2	3	4
5	6	7	8	9	10	11
12	13	14	15	16	17	18
19	20	21	22	23	24	25
26	27	28	29	30	31	

August
S	M	T	W	T	F	S
						1
2	3	4	5	6	7	8
9	10	11	12	13	14	15
16	17	18	19	20	21	22
23	24	25	26	27	28	29
30	31					

September
S	M	T	W	T	F	S
		1	2	3	4	5
6	7	8	9	10	11	12
13	14	15	16	17	18	19
20	21	22	23	24	25	26
27	28	29	30			

October
S	M	T	W	T	F	S
				1	2	3
4	5	6	7	8	9	10
11	12	13	14	15	16	17
18	19	20	21	22	23	24
25	26	27	28	29	30	31

November
S	M	T	W	T	F	S
1	2	3	4	5	6	7
8	9	10	11	12	13	14
15	16	17	18	19	20	21
22	23	24	25	26	27	28
29	30					

December
S	M	T	W	T	F	S
		1	2	3	4	5
6	7	8	9	10	11	12
13	14	15	16	17	18	19
20	21	22	23	24	25	26
27	28	29	30	31		

2022

January
S	M	T	W	T	F	S
						1
2	3	4	5	6	7	8
9	10	11	12	13	14	15
16	17	18	19	20	21	22
23	24	25	26	27	28	29
30	31					

February
S	M	T	W	T	F	S
		1	2	3	4	5
6	7	8	9	10	11	12
13	14	15	16	17	18	19
20	21	22	23	24	25	26
27	28					

March
S	M	T	W	T	F	S
		1	2	3	4	5
6	7	8	9	10	11	12
13	14	15	16	17	18	19
20	21	22	23	24	25	26
27	28	29	30	31		

April
S	M	T	W	T	F	S
					1	2
3	4	5	6	7	8	9
10	11	12	13	14	15	16
17	18	19	20	21	22	23
24	25	26	27	28	29	30

May
S	M	T	W	T	F	S
1	2	3	4	5	6	7
8	9	10	11	12	13	14
15	16	17	18	19	20	21
22	23	24	25	26	27	28
29	30	31				

June
S	M	T	W	T	F	S
			1	2	3	4
5	6	7	8	9	10	11
12	13	14	15	16	17	18
19	20	21	22	23	24	25
26	27	28	29	30		

July
S	M	T	W	T	F	S
					1	2
3	4	5	6	7	8	9
10	11	12	13	14	15	16
17	18	19	20	21	22	23
24	25	26	27	28	29	30
31						

August
S	M	T	W	T	F	S
	1	2	3	4	5	6
7	8	9	10	11	12	13
14	15	16	17	18	19	20
21	22	23	24	25	26	27
28	29	30	31			

September
S	M	T	W	T	F	S
				1	2	3
4	5	6	7	8	9	10
11	12	13	14	15	16	17
18	19	20	21	22	23	24
25	26	27	28	29	30	

October
S	M	T	W	T	F	S
						1
2	3	4	5	6	7	8
9	10	11	12	13	14	15
16	17	18	19	20	21	22
23	24	25	26	27	28	29
30	31					

November
S	M	T	W	T	F	S
		1	2	3	4	5
6	7	8	9	10	11	12
13	14	15	16	17	18	19
20	21	22	23	24	25	26
27	28	29	30			

December
S	M	T	W	T	F	S
				1	2	3
4	5	6	7	8	9	10
11	12	13	14	15	16	17
18	19	20	21	22	23	24
25	26	27	28	29	30	31

2021

January

S	M	T	W	T	F	S
					1	2
3	4	5	6	7	8	9
10	11	12	13	14	15	16
17	18	19	20	21	22	23
24	25	26	27	28	29	30
31						

February

S	M	T	W	T	F	S
	1	2	3	4	5	6
7	8	9	10	11	12	13
14	15	16	17	18	19	20
21	22	23	24	25	26	27
28						

March

S	M	T	W	T	F	S
	1	2	3	4	5	6
7	8	9	10	11	12	13
14	15	16	17	18	19	20
21	22	23	24	25	26	27
28	29	30	31			

April

S	M	T	W	T	F	S
				1	2	3
4	5	6	7	8	9	10
11	12	13	14	15	16	17
18	19	20	21	22	23	24
25	26	27	28	29	30	

May

S	M	T	W	T	F	S
						1
2	3	4	5	6	7	8
9	10	11	12	13	14	15
16	17	18	19	20	21	22
23	24	25	26	27	28	29
30	31					

June

S	M	T	W	T	F	S
		1	2	3	4	5
6	7	8	9	10	11	12
13	14	15	16	17	18	19
20	21	22	23	24	25	26
27	28	29	30			

July

S	M	T	W	T	F	S
				1	2	3
4	5	6	7	8	9	10
11	12	13	14	15	16	17
18	19	20	21	22	23	24
25	26	27	28	29	30	31

August

S	M	T	W	T	F	S
1	2	3	4	5	6	7
8	9	10	11	12	13	14
15	16	17	18	19	20	21
22	23	24	25	26	27	28
29	30	31				

September

S	M	T	W	T	F	S
			1	2	3	4
5	6	7	8	9	10	11
12	13	14	15	16	17	18
19	20	21	22	23	24	25
26	27	28	29	30		

October

S	M	T	W	T	F	S
					1	2
3	4	5	6	7	8	9
10	11	12	13	14	15	16
17	18	19	20	21	22	23
24	25	26	27	28	29	30
31						

November

S	M	T	W	T	F	S
	1	2	3	4	5	6
7	8	9	10	11	12	13
14	15	16	17	18	19	20
21	22	23	24	25	26	27
28	29	30				

December

S	M	T	W	T	F	S
			1	2	3	4
5	6	7	8	9	10	11
12	13	14	15	16	17	18
19	20	21	22	23	24	25
26	27	28	29	30	31	

INTRODUCTION

Can you outrun your own biology? This is one of many thorny questions runners had to confront in the past year. Also, who counts as a woman? Why are distance races without finish lines surging in appeal? Are you racing against a competitor or against a shoe technology? You'd believe that track and field was coming apart. As these matters settle themselves, try to see the opportunities to change your own training program this year. Even if you have no interest in competition, elite runners are showing the way to see yourself and your running abilities in entirely new ways. They may not revolutionize your workouts. But they can help you redefine your goals.

Courtney Dauwalter loves to kick men's butts . . . on the occasions that she sees them at all. The 34-year-old former science teacher is usually too far in front of the pack—by as much as ten hours in the case of the Moab 240 Endurance Run (Dauwalter's finishing time: 2 days, 9 hours, 59 minutes). She is the first woman to win Steamboat Springs' Run Rabbit Run, a 100-miler with 20,000 feet elevation up and down. She has won more than 32 ultra-events and has been known to go so hard that she actually lost her eyesight for the last 12 miles in one race.

The topic of ultramarathon running usually arises with the words "lunacy," "obsessive," or "nihilistic" kicking into conversation, and these merely describe the motivations of competitors. The physiology for running such distances can't be explained at all. There are no training rules, no accepted methods of coaching. Science is at a loss to show any discernible patterns in metabolism that allow humans to run such astonishing distances. And the inherent advantages of gender seem to disappear after the first 50 miles or so.

Dauwalter sticks to a "no-plan plan" for races, eating everything from McDonald's double cheeseburgers and Tailwind nutrition snacks to mashed potatoes. Nor does she train with any organized rigor, believing simply that as her threshold for pain increases, she can run farther. Can a runner's psychological fortitude prevail over muscle mass and size? This year, why not find out for yourself?

Charles Allie plans to do just that. You are in a rare class of athletes if you can run 400 meters in less than one minute, even if you are a teenage track star. Allie was 71 when he broke his own world record at 57.26 seconds in 2017. The Pittsburgh native has been beating the one-minute mark since he began winning city championships in high school. Today he sails past his own age cohort by 30 or 40 meters. He also holds the world record for 200 meters. And in an eye-popping dare to Father Time, he plans to beat the record for 100 meters in his age group, which would make him the only Masters Runner ever to hold three world records.

From your mid-20s on, athletic performance declines about 6 percent each decade. That's the trajectory for an average body. Add injuries, youthful lifestyle assaults to your cardiovascular system, osteoarthritis, poundage come and gone (sometimes come again), and the downward slope steepens. Allie began running sub-minute 400s when the first health warnings on cigarettes appeared, the skateboard came into vogue, and the Beatles topped the AM radio play charts. He stayed normally healthy, trained moderately, and has run the Penn Relays every year since he was 40. Given the broad spectrum of injuries that sprinters are prone to, Allie's slow descent is remarkable. Not even he can say how much of his gift he owes to genetic luck.

In all likelihood, you can't say much about your own. High school coaches may have spotted a middle-distance runner in your physique or a cross-country star. You can find some clues about your abilities in the bodies of your parents, especially if they were runners, but also in the uneven ways that aging insinuates itself into their postures, body weight, and stride. Unfortunately, biological clues and ability don't always agree.

Even though she had won an athletic scholarship, Allie Kieffer never "looked" like a champion runner—and was reminded by it at every turn. "You could lose five pounds," she was told, regardless of what her current weight was (today she is 5'4", 120 lb.). In message chains and social media, scoldings from coaches, and slurs from competitors, she felt an endless drumbeat to lose weight. So she did. And then she lost more, and her body finally revolted. She quit running altogether.

After college, she moved from Boulder to New York and slowly reconnected to her old passion— but entirely on her own terms. There were no goals, no racing, and no coaches. She jogged in Central Park with friends and joined a CrossFit gym. She got faster—much faster. At the 2017 New York City Marathon, Kieffer placed fifth (2:29:39). In 2018, she placed seventh (2:28:12). Today the 33-year-old is a coach and nutritionist. For runners everywhere, she represents the power of shrugging off preconceived notions about how to achieve your goals. This year, instead of obsessing about your inadequacies, build on your strengths. An entirely different kind of champion may emerge.

Even ancient measures for track and field victories are evolving. Running competition has traditionally been divided by gender, originally determined by what was apparent to the eye, but now defined by a runner's chromosomes—or to testosterone levels and how the body responds to them. Less than a year after India's supreme court overturned a ban on gay sex, Dutee Chand won the right to race against other women, even though she has hyperandrogenism, a condition that naturally produces high testosterone levels. Guinness World Records now include 78 titles for the marathon, including the fastest times for a runner in a wedding dress, dressed as a dragon, or in the disguise of an astronomical body. So this year, set your goals accordingly.

—**Marty Jerome** ◼

January 2021

SUNDAY	MONDAY	TUESDAY	WEDNESDAY	THURSDAY	FRIDAY	SATURDAY
					1	2
					New Year's Day Kwanzaa ends (USA)	
3	4	5	6	7	8	9
	New Year's Day (observed) (NZ) Bank Holiday (UK—Scotland)					
10	11	12	13	14	15	16
17	18	19	20	21	22	23
	Martin Luther King Jr. Day (USA)					
24	25	26	27	28	29	30
31		Australia Day				

"Be willing to be a beginner every single morning."

—Meister Eckhart

SPEAK

The next time running comes up in conversation, listen to how you talk about it. Poetic or technical, adjectives or verbs, language captures only part of the experience and almost never the personal part. Likely, words aren't what fail you. Most runners speak about goals or achievements instead of purpose, as if *what* could explain *why*. To get more from your workouts this year, flip the conversation. Listen to what running says about *you*.

That you train at all proves you believe personal change is possible and that you have some control over its direction. When you were new to running, this required a leap of faith. Does this gutsiness show up in other parts of your life—say, your ease at taking on a large home-improvement project or your instincts for striking up a conversation with an attractive stranger? When psychological risk fades from a training program, progress is doomed. Find ways to dare yourself, even in the smallest daily decisions, then watch how this habit of mind helps you get more from your workouts.

Running doesn't necessarily signal that you're an insufferably rigid detail freak, but it hints that you prefer order over chaos. After all, a training program is basically just organized effort, the more organized, the better the results. Just make sure consistency doesn't turn you into a monster. If you're horrified when a work colleague asks to accompany you on a run or enraged when a trail closure forces you to an unfamiliar route, your workouts might need fresh perspective (or your diet needs more fiber). Mental flexibility isn't just an accommodation to the messy demands of daily living. It makes you a better runner, forcing you to resort priorities on the fly, broaden goals, reimagine payoffs, and enjoy the ride. A workout cancelled because of a lightning storm can be downright therapeutic.

Runners have a peculiar, sometimes fetishistic relationship with numbers. Whatever your goals, numerals are short answers to the long question posed by dedicated exertion, whether they tick from a stopwatch or glare at you from a bathroom scale. You can't argue with them. Remind yourself that the runner, not the number, is the sheriff of your training program. If the level of effort feels right and your commitment to training is both reasonable and satisfying, disappointing tallies suggest your goals are off. Go find some new numbers.

Even your running form reveals your essential character. You can read focus and intent from hips and arm swing. Feet slapping the ground indicate that fatigue is pushing in. Are you the kind of person who denies the pain or wears it with defiance? As in life, tears can mean anything, though they're sometimes accompanied by a humble sadness that sweeps across the face when a victory is nigh. And there is nothing more exultant and personally revealing than the last few strides of a runner who has spent absolutely everything within. It's a great reminder that talk is cheap. ∎

Distance carried forward: _____

28 Monday
_____
_____
_____

Where & When: _____ Distance: _____
Comments: _____
_____

29 Tuesday
_____
_____
_____

Where & When: _____ Distance: _____
Comments: _____
_____

30 Wednesday
_____
_____
_____

Where & When: _____ Distance: _____
Comments: _____
_____

31 Thursday
_____
_____
_____

Where & When: _____ Distance: _____
Comments: _____
_____

1 Friday
1
_____
_____

Where & When: _____ Distance: _____
Comments: _____
_____

Dec 2020/Jan

Saturday 2

Where & When: _____   Distance: _____

Comments: _____

Sunday 3

Where & When: _____   Distance: _____

Comments: _____

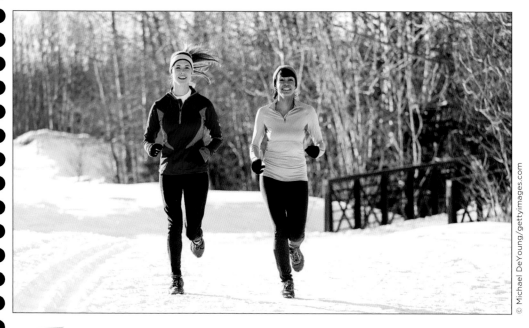

© Michael DeYoung/gettyimages.com

tip: Don't overthink your running form. Over time and miles, your body will generally find the most efficient way to move.

Distance this week: _____   Weight: _____

Distance carried forward:

4 Monday   4

Where & When: Distance:

Comments:

5 Tuesday   5

Where & When: Distance:

Comments:

6 Wednesday   6

Where & When: Distance:

Comments:

7 Thursday   7

Where & When: Distance:

Comments:

8 Friday   8

Where & When: Distance:

Comments:

January

9

Where & When: _____ Distance: _____

Comments: _____

10 **Sunday 10**

Where & When: _____ Distance: _____

Comments: _____

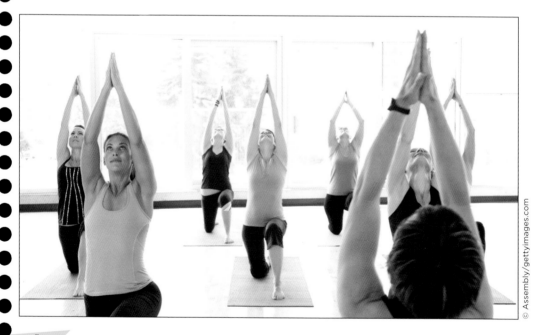

© Assembly/gettyimages.com

tip: Chronic lower back pain? Try yoga. Studies show that it can be as effective as physical therapy for relieving agony.

Distance this week: _____ **Weight:** _____

Distance carried forward: _____

11 Monday   11

_____
_____
_____

Where & When: _____ **Distance:** _____

Comments: _____
_____

12 Tuesday   12

_____
_____
_____

Where & When: _____ **Distance:** _____

Comments: _____
_____

13 Wednesday   13

_____
_____
_____

Where & When: _____ **Distance:** _____

Comments: _____
_____

14 Thursday   14

_____
_____
_____

Where & When: _____ **Distance:** _____

Comments: _____
_____

15 Friday   15

_____
_____
_____

Where & When: _____ **Distance:** _____

Comments: _____
_____

January

Saturday 16

16

Where & When: _____ Distance: _____

Comments: _____

Sunday 17

17

Where & When: _____ Distance: _____

Comments: _____

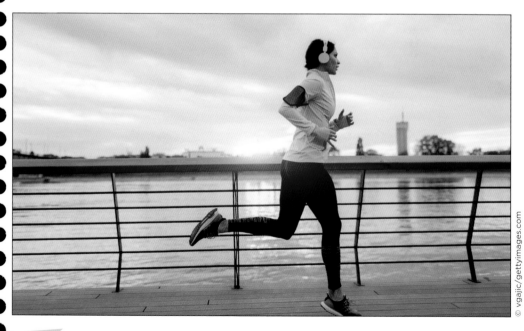

© vgajic/gettyimages.com

tip: A good workout headset does *not* cancel ambient sounds.

Distance this week: _____ Weight: _____

Distance carried forward: _____

18 Monday   18

_____

_____

Where & When: _____ **Distance:** _____

Comments: _____

19 Tuesday   19

_____

_____

Where & When: _____ **Distance:** _____

Comments: _____

20 Wednesday   20

_____

_____

Where & When: _____ **Distance:** _____

Comments: _____

21 Thursday   21

_____

_____

Where & When: _____ **Distance:** _____

Comments: _____

22 Friday   22

_____

_____

Where & When: _____ **Distance:** _____

Comments: _____

January

Saturday 23

23

Where & When: _____   Distance: _____

Comments: _____

Sunday 24

24

Where & When: _____   Distance: _____

Comments: _____

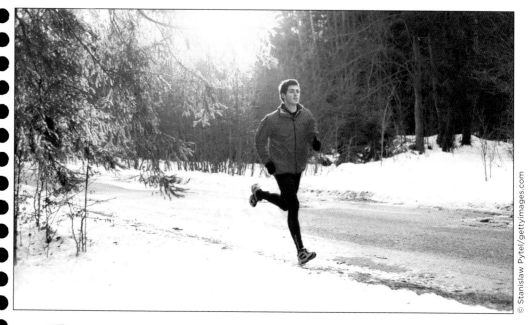

© Stanislaw Pytel/gettyimages.com

tip: For all its many health benefits, running does *not* offset the metabolic ills caused by sedentary living, including diabetes and heart disease.

Distance this week: _____   Weight: _____

Distance carried forward: _____

25 Monday 25

_____
_____
_____

Where & When: _____ **Distance:** _____
Comments: _____

26 Tuesday 26

_____
_____
_____

Where & When: _____ **Distance:** _____
Comments: _____

27 Wednesday 27

_____
_____
_____

Where & When: _____ **Distance:** _____
Comments: _____

28 Thursday 28

_____
_____
_____

Where & When: _____ **Distance:** _____
Comments: _____

29 Friday 29

_____
_____
_____

Where & When: _____ **Distance:** _____
Comments: _____

January

Saturday 30

30

Where & When: _____ Distance: _____

Comments: _____

Sunday 31

31

Where & When: _____ Distance: _____

Comments: _____

"Only the strong appreciate the warmth emanating from those who can turn obstacles into fuel."
—Garry Fitchett

tip: Company wellness programs do little to lower employee cholesterol or sugar levels, or any other measures of general health. Use them to augment—not replace—your own training.

Notes: _____

Distance this week: _____ Weight: _____

February 2021

SUNDAY	MONDAY	TUESDAY	WEDNESDAY	THURSDAY	FRIDAY	SATURDAY
	1	2	3	4	5	6
						Waitangi Day (NZ)
7	8	9	10	11	12	13
	Waitangi Day (observed) (NZ)					
14	15	16	17	18	19	20
St. Valentine's Day	Presidents' Day (USA)		Ash Wednesday			
21	22	23	24	25	26	27
					Purim*	
28						

*Begins at sundown the previous day

"We are made to persist. That's how we find out who we are."
—Tobias Wolff

WIMP

Think you're tough? Sure, you're strong. You feel your strength in every step, in every tug of your hamstrings. It's the same with courage, which you test in countless ways, beginning with the first time you laced up running shoes. But toughness is different; indispensable to any runner, but mysterious in how much you can actually call on; unreliable in how long you can sustain it, and difficult to prevent from careening into recklessness. It lies to you, and still you need it. Can you train to be tough?

First dispense with heroic images of yourself with mud-smeared thighs and tears streaming down your grinning face, that sort of thing. You don't need tights and a cape to prove you're tough, and these ideas will only get you into trouble. When your mind says yes but your body says no, there's usually room for negotiation, but it has to start quickly, sometimes within a matter of strides. Weak runners react. The rugged decide. Finding clarity of mind under extreme stress comes naturally to very few runners. For the rest of us, endurance training helps. So does trail running. Meanwhile, in the moment of anguish, learn to focus on the facts your body telegraphs, not how you feel about them or what they portend. Emotions are the first thing to dump.

Pain muddies matters because it conveys both fact and feeling, so try to keep these separate. Most of us can work through muscle cramps and the first dispiriting waves of fatigue. Instead of ignoring or wishing these away, begin a conversation with yourself. Even saying aloud, "This hurts," puts pain in a mental box, separate from what your body is trying to accomplish. It stops a full-on freak-out, what psychologists call catastrophizing, allowing you to monitor the progress of your misery like a forest ranger from a fire tower. For runners, toughness is mostly about patient vigilance.

If all this sounds a little Zen-like smug when sweat and sometimes blood are very tangible parts of your predicament, bear in mind that meditation is now a common part of training for elite athletes. So are mantras: "Commit, then figure it out," "Feelings can wait," "You'll cherish the memory," or "All things will pass." Find your own chants and prayers to help you persist to the end. Mantras aren't just incantations about personal resolve. They prepare you for bad situations that might turn worse.

Indeed, preparation is a form of toughness, surprise its foil. Anyone who has run the Boston Marathon knows that Heartbreak Hill gets its name for a reason, but at least you know it's coming. A twisted ankle from loose gravel or sudden intestinal distress throws everything into chaos. Should you visualize a finish line, a porta potty, or an ambulance? Toughness won't help you here, nor mantras, and it's important to know their limitations. They're not superpowers. But when you need to make a decision you don't want to make, they sometimes bring clarity and sometimes peace because tough runners sometimes quit. They also cry. ∎

Distance carried forward:

1 Monday 32

Where & When: _____ Distance: _____

Comments:

2 Tuesday 33

Where & When: _____ Distance: _____

Comments:

3 Wednesday 34

Where & When: _____ Distance: _____

Comments:

4 Thursday 35

Where & When: _____ Distance: _____

Comments:

5 Friday 36

Where & When: _____ Distance: _____

Comments:

February

Saturday 6

Where & When: _____ Distance: _____

Comments: _____

Sunday 7

Where & When: _____ Distance: _____

Comments: _____

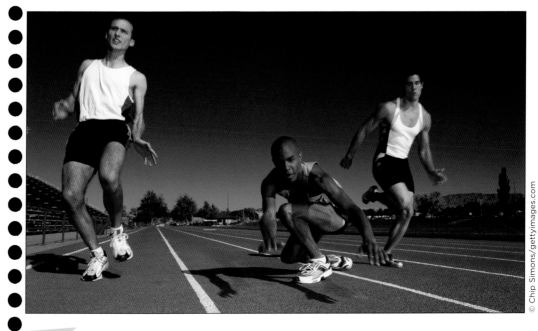

© Chip Simons/gettyimages.com

tip: When a fall is unstoppable, throw your hands out to protect your head and face, but don't stiffen your elbows.

Distance this week: _____ Weight: _____

Distance carried forward: _____

8 Monday 39

_____
_____

Where & When: _____ **Distance:** _____
Comments: _____
_____

9 Tuesday 40

_____
_____

Where & When: _____ **Distance:** _____
Comments: _____
_____

10 Wednesday 41

_____
_____

Where & When: _____ **Distance:** _____
Comments: _____
_____

11 Thursday 42

_____
_____

Where & When: _____ **Distance:** _____
Comments: _____
_____

12 Friday 43

_____
_____

Where & When: _____ **Distance:** _____
Comments: _____

February

Saturday 13

44

Where & When: _____ Distance: _____

Comments: _____

Sunday 14

45

Where & When: _____ Distance: _____

Comments: _____

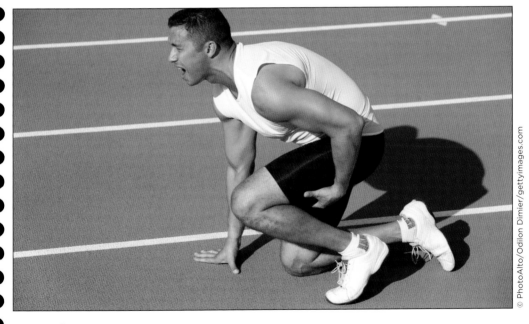

© PhotoAlto/Odilon Dimier/gettyimages.com

tip: Suck it up for pain. Ibuprofen and other nonsteroidal anti-inflammatory drugs (NSAIDs) may overtax the kidneys during prolonged exercise and reduce muscles' ability to recover afterward.

Distance this week: _____ **Weight:** _____

Distance carried forward: _____

15 Monday
46
_____
_____

Where & When: _____ **Distance:** _____
Comments: _____
_____

16 Tuesday
47
_____
_____

Where & When: _____ **Distance:** _____
Comments: _____
_____

17 Wednesday
48
_____
_____

Where & When: _____ **Distance:** _____
Comments: _____
_____

18 Thursday
49
_____
_____

Where & When: _____ **Distance:** _____
Comments: _____
_____

19 Friday
50
_____
_____

Where & When: _____ **Distance:** _____
Comments: _____
_____

February

51

Where & When: _____ Distance: _____

Comments: _____

52

Where & When: _____ Distance: _____

Comments: _____

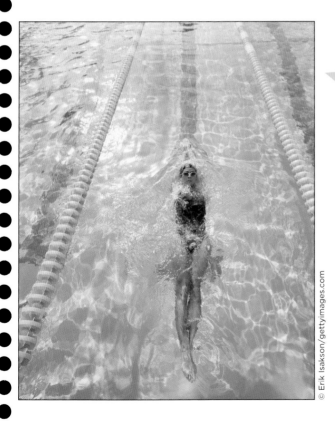

© Erik Isakson/gettyimages.com

tip: Swimming may alleviate some back pain caused by running. The breast- and backstrokes are recommended because they don't hyperextend back muscles.

Distance this week: _____ Weight: _____

22 Monday
53

Where & When: **Distance:**

Comments:

23 Tuesday
54

Where & When: **Distance:**

Comments:

24 Wednesday
55

Where & When: **Distance:**

Comments:

25 Thursday
56

Where & When: **Distance:**

Comments:

26 Friday
57

Where & When: **Distance:**

Comments:

February

58

Where & When: Distance:

Comments:

59   Sunday 28

Where & When: Distance:

Comments:

"You may not control all the events that happen to you, but you can decide not to be reduced by them."

—Maya Angelou

tip: Remember your comebacks—whether from injury, failure, or misfortune. They are vital memories to a training program when spirits or progress begin to flag.

Notes:

Distance this week: Weight:

March 2021

SUNDAY	MONDAY	TUESDAY	WEDNESDAY	THURSDAY	FRIDAY	SATURDAY
	1 St. David's Day (UK) Labour Day (Australia—WA)	2	3	4	5	6
7	8 International Women's Day Eight Hours Day (Australia—TAS) Canberra Day (Australia—ACT) Labour Day (Australia—VIC) Commonwealth Day (Australia, Canada, NZ, UK)	9	10	11	12	13
14 Mothering Sunday (Ireland, UK)	15	16	17 St. Patrick's Day	18	19	20
21	22	23	24	25	26	27
28 Palm Sunday Passover*	29	30	31			

*Begins at sundown the previous day

"*Turn your wounds into wisdom.*"
—Oprah Winfrey

FRENEMIES

Right Knee: "You're at it again. I told you this wasn't a day for hill charges, but did you listen? Would an easy distance workout have killed you for one more day while I recover?"

You: "Sorry. I thought a slow warm-up would put you in the mood . . . I guess I overestimated.

Left Knee: "Oh, listen to Right Knee—always the complainer, that one. I carry just as much of the load, but do you hear me griping about a little elevation, a little hard work?"

Right Knee: "Who needs to gripe with all the popping and grinding noises you make. What's up with that? You sound like the rigging on an old mule wagon. It scares us, you know that, right? It makes us think one day you're going to give out flat."

Left Knee: "I'm not pampered like you are, what with the compression sleeve—there's not one bit of evidence those things actually work, do you know that? They look ridiculous. You get the post-shower bag of frozen peas. Do I get the frozen peas? No, I do not."

You: "I love and respect both of my knees equally, but I try to attend to your individual needs."

Right Knee: "They always say that, but it's never true. If you really loved us equally, you'd get Quadriceps to pick up more of the work on hills, especially downslopes, instead of lying around like mashed potatoes on a school kid's lunch plate. Hey, Quads, try a few squats maybe. Hop on the leg press."

Left Knee: "Share the love, Quads! Share the pain! We're not feeling it over here!"

You: "I should probably spend more time stretching Calves as well."

Left Knee: "Calves, Calves! Those showboats cause trouble all the way up Hips to Back and Neck."

Right Knee: "Yeah, Back is a moaner. It's disgusting."

Left Knee: "You want to really do everyone a favor? Stop two-timing us with tarted-up street shoes. Heels, Italian oxfords—you spend half the day in flip-flops! Get some decent footwear with arch support.

You: "I'll lose the flip-flops."

Right Knee: "While you're at it, lose the attitude. We could use a little attention down here. Stop treating us like we're cheap labor. A night out would be nice. How about an evening of hip flexor stretches, leg lifts, standing calf stretches, and sultry wall slides? Sound relaxing? That is, unless Left Knee brings the squeaky orchestra—the Pops. A total mood killer."

Left Knee: "You should be chained to a treadmill."

Right Knee: "Maybe a little party right before bedtime, yeah? But easy on the ibuprofen. Not good for the kidneys."

You: "I'll think about it."

Left Knee: "Hey, have you noticed that Butt is getting bigger?"

Right Knee: "Yeah, but don't say anything. Butt is sensitive." ∎

Distance carried forward: _____

1 Monday 60

_____
_____
_____

Where & When: _____ **Distance:** _____
Comments: _____

2 Tuesday 61

_____
_____
_____

Where & When: _____ **Distance:** _____
Comments: _____

3 Wednesday 62

_____
_____
_____

Where & When: _____ **Distance:** _____
Comments: _____

4 Thursday 63

_____
_____
_____

Where & When: _____ **Distance:** _____
Comments: _____

5 Friday 64

_____
_____
_____

Where & When: _____ **Distance:** _____
Comments: _____

March

Where & When: Distance:

Comments:

Where & When: Distance:

Comments:

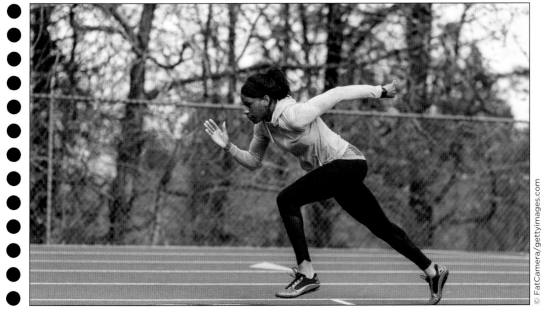

© FatCamera/gettyimages.com

tip: The best one-minute intervals for runners who hate intervals is called 10-20-30. Go slow for 30 seconds, a moderate pace for 20 seconds, and then a hard sprint for 10 seconds. They're easy (and addictive).

Distance this week: **Weight:**

Distance carried forward: _____

8 Monday   67
_____
_____
_____

Where & When: _____ **Distance:** _____
Comments: _____
_____

9 Tuesday   68
_____
_____
_____

Where & When: _____ **Distance:** _____
Comments: _____
_____

10 Wednesday   69
_____
_____
_____

Where & When: _____ **Distance:** _____
Comments: _____
_____

11 Thursday   70
_____
_____
_____

Where & When: _____ **Distance:** _____
Comments: _____
_____

12 Friday   71
_____
_____
_____

Where & When: _____ **Distance:** _____
Comments: _____
_____

March

Saturday 13

Where & When: _____ Distance: _____

Comments: _____

Sunday 14

Where & When: _____ Distance: _____

Comments: _____

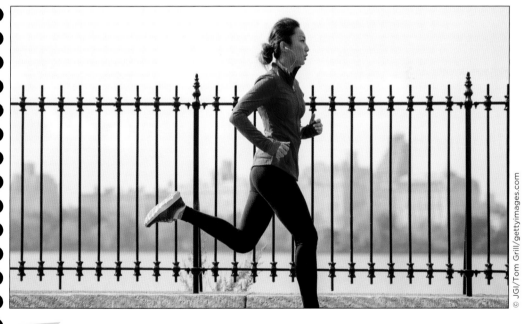

© JGI/Tom Grill/gettyimages.com

tip: Women runners suffer fewer injuries than men probably because they have a shorter stride.

Distance this week: _____ **Weight:** _____

Distance carried forward: _____

15 Monday 74

_____
_____

Where & When: _____ **Distance:** _____
Comments: _____

_____

16 Tuesday 75

_____
_____

Where & When: _____ **Distance:** _____
Comments: _____

_____

17 Wednesday 76

_____
_____

Where & When: _____ **Distance:** _____
Comments: _____

_____

18 Thursday 77

_____
_____

Where & When: _____ **Distance:** _____
Comments: _____

_____

19 Friday 78

_____
_____

Where & When: _____ **Distance:** _____
Comments: _____

_____

March

Saturday 20

79

Where & When: _____ **Distance:** _____
Comments: _____

Sunday 21

80

Where & When: _____ **Distance:** _____
Comments: _____

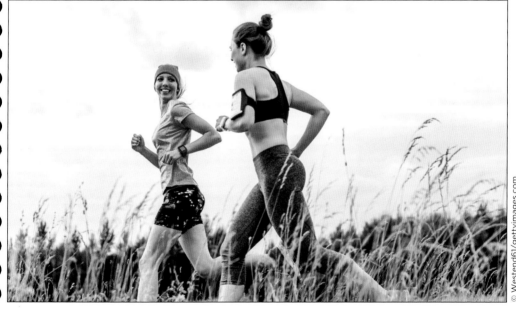

© Westend61/gettyimages.com

tip: Sorry, guys, but women generally pace themselves better in distance races.

Distance this week: _____ **Weight:** _____

Distance carried forward:

22 Monday   81

Where & When: Distance:
Comments:

23 Tuesday   82

Where & When: Distance:
Comments:

24 Wednesday   83

Where & When: Distance:
Comments:

25 Thursday   84

Where & When: Distance:
Comments:

26 Friday   85

Where & When: Distance:
Comments:

March

Saturday 27

Where & When: _____ Distance: _____

Comments: _____

Sunday 28

Where & When: _____ Distance: _____

Comments: _____

"Perfection is not attainable, but if we chase perfection we can catch excellence."
—Vince Lombardi

tip: Heating pads might be soothing, but they're useless for speeding recovery from an injury.

Notes: _____

Distance this week: _____ Weight: _____

April 2021

SUNDAY	MONDAY	TUESDAY	WEDNESDAY	THURSDAY	FRIDAY	SATURDAY
				1	**2** Good Friday (Western)	**3** Easter Saturday (Australia—except TAS, WA)
4 Easter (Western) Passover ends	**5** Easter Monday (Australia, Canada, Ireland, NZ, UK—except Scotland)	**6**	**7**	**8**	**9**	**10**
11	**12** Ramadan	**13**	**14**	**15**	**16**	**17**
18	**19**	**20**	**21**	**22** Earth Day	**23** St. George's Day (UK)	**24**
25 Anzac Day (NZ, Australia)	**26** Anzac Day (observed) (NZ, Australia—ACT, SA, WA)	**27**	**28**	**29**	**30** Holy Friday (Orthodox)	

"You can't win unless you learn how to lose."

—Kareem Abdul-Jabbar

CHICKEN

A race registration form should scare you. It should threaten some primitive and personal conception you hold about yourself, even your place in the cosmic order. Your nervousness—even terror—proves that the event has slipped past the tripwires and barricades of your imagination, that it has seen sufficient daylight so as to become an actual possibility. If you're not afraid of the entry form, you've picked the wrong race. Otherwise, sign your name.

Are you hesitating? If it's your first marathon or if you're returning to competition after a long time down, the stakes are psychologically higher than you might appreciate. So consider what failure would mean to you. This may require you to rearrange the way you hold the event in your mind or what you hope to accomplish by competing in it. At least you'll face it aware, and this is a kind of fortitude. It should shoo away your hesitancy even if it does nothing for your split times.

Next consider what's holding you back from a race. It's easy enough to list the logistical snares, from calendar conflicts to costs and the time it takes to reach a competitive level, even factoring in an unforeseen bout with a cold or a relationship gone kablooey. List only the tangible obstacles. Leave aside self-doubt, flatline enthusiasm, romantic distractions, and arthritis that comes and goes. Most problems that stand in your way to a starting line have a number attached to them. Can you work around them or draw them down to zero?

Now talk to people, especially those who couldn't care less about whether you enter a running competition. As the Buddha might have observed, they have beginner's minds. They will ask questions and offer advice you won't hear from your running partner, your spouse, or your dog. Consult those beings as well, but only under the condition that their counsel will be dispassionate and practical and that you will love them no less for what they tell you. Yes, lie to them.

Return to numbers. However you measure your progress, read not too much, nor too little from the miles, seconds, pounds, finishes, and dusty trophies you have shaved or accumulated. Nevertheless, your training history is your guide to future events, and its language is numerals. Study them. Count the weeks until race day, and plot as if training in a perfect universe without interruptions and setbacks. Ask the numerals if your race is doable, and regardless of the answer, end the conversation.

Cheat. Runners everywhere and at every level celebrate the signing of a race-entry form as an official covenant of commitment, kind of like a bris. Runners bring the wrong mindset to it. For your next race, drop the form into the mailbox, and tell no one you did it. Just start training. When your progress reaches a level that signals you made the right decision, then go ahead and blab. You will be accused of holding out, even deception. Feh. They will love you no less. ■

Distance carried forward: _____

29 Monday 88

_____

_____

_____

Where & When: _____ Distance: _____

Comments: _____

30 Tuesday 89

_____

_____

_____

Where & When: _____ Distance: _____

Comments: _____

31 Wednesday 90

_____

_____

_____

Where & When: _____ Distance: _____

Comments: _____

1 Thursday 91

_____

_____

_____

Where & When: _____ Distance: _____

Comments: _____

2 Friday 92

_____

_____

_____

Where & When: _____ Distance: _____

Comments: _____

March/April

Saturday 3

Where & When: _____ Distance: _____

Comments: _____

Sunday 4

Where & When: _____ Distance: _____

Comments: _____

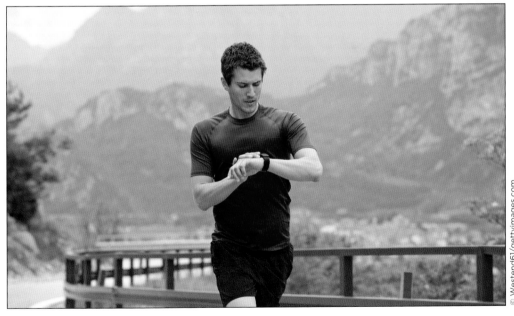

© Westend61/gettyimages.com

tip: Run-walk workouts are excellent if you're returning. Time the beginning and duration of walk breaks. Don't just walk when you're tired.

Distance this week: _____ Weight: _____

Distance carried forward: _____

5 Monday

95

_____
_____

Where & When: _____ **Distance:** _____
Comments:
_____

6 Tuesday

96

_____
_____

Where & When: _____ **Distance:** _____
Comments:
_____

7 Wednesday

97

_____
_____

Where & When: _____ **Distance:** _____
Comments:
_____

8 Thursday

98

_____
_____

Where & When: _____ **Distance:** _____
Comments:
_____

9 Friday

99

_____
_____

Where & When: _____ **Distance:** _____
Comments:
_____

April

Saturday 10

100

Where & When: _____ Distance: _____

Comments: _____

Sunday 11

101

Where & When: _____ Distance: _____

Comments: _____

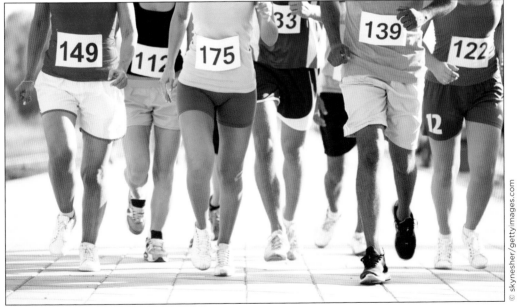

© skynesher/gettyimages.com

tip: In planning your next marathon, calculate your average mile pace from your last marathon to use as a benchmark. Also examine your pace at various stages of the race.

Distance this week: _____ Weight: _____

Distance carried forward:

12 Monday 102

Where & When: **Distance:**

Comments:

13 Tuesday 103

Where & When: **Distance:**

Comments:

14 Wednesday 104

Where & When: **Distance:**

Comments:

15 Thursday 105

Where & When: **Distance:**

Comments:

16 Friday 106

Where & When: **Distance:**

Comments:

Saturday 17

107

_____

_____

_____

Where & When: _____ **Distance:** _____

Comments: _____

Sunday 18

108

_____

_____

_____

Where & When: _____ **Distance:** _____

Comments: _____

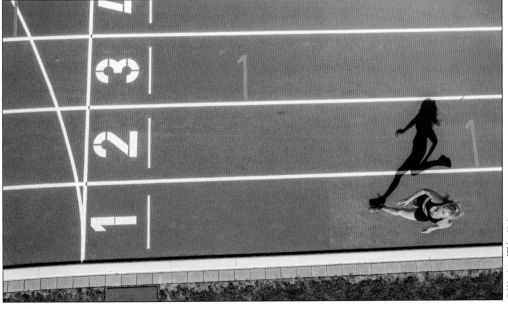

© Westend61/gettyimages.com

tip: Don't dismiss the value of rehearsal races leading up to a big event. They prepare you for crowds, the effects of weather on performance, the ways that pacing can be thrown off, and toilet breaks.

Distance this week: _____ **Weight:** _____

Distance carried forward: _____

19 Monday   109

_____
_____
_____

Where & When: _____ **Distance:** _____
Comments: _____
_____

20 Tuesday   110

_____
_____
_____

Where & When: _____ **Distance:** _____
Comments: _____
_____

21 Wednesday   111

_____
_____
_____

Where & When: _____ **Distance:** _____
Comments: _____
_____

22 Thursday   112

_____
_____
_____

Where & When: _____ **Distance:** _____
Comments: _____
_____

23 Friday   113

_____
_____
_____

Where & When: _____ **Distance:** _____
Comments: _____
_____

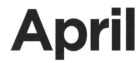

114 _____

_____

_____

Where & When: _____ **Distance:** _____

Comments: _____

_____

115 _____ **Sunday 25**

_____

_____

Where & When: _____ **Distance:** _____

Comments: _____

_____

"Always be a first-rate version of yourself instead of a second-rate version of someone else."
—Judy Garland

tip: Though the evidence keeps shifting, the best studies to date show that those who skip breakfast are more likely to be obese and have high cholesterol.

Notes: _____

_____

_____

_____

_____

Distance this week: _____ **Weight:** _____

May 2021

SUNDAY	MONDAY	TUESDAY	WEDNESDAY	THURSDAY	FRIDAY	SATURDAY
						1
2 Easter (Orthodox)	**3** May Day (Australia—NT) Labour Day (Australia—QLD) Early May Bank Holiday (Ireland, UK)	**4**	**5**	**6**	**7**	**8**
9 Mother's Day (USA, Australia, Canada, NZ)	**10**	**11**	**12** Eid al-Fitr	**13**	**14**	**15** Armed Forces Day (USA)
16	**17**	**18**	**19**	**20**	**21**	**22**
23	**24** Victoria Day (Canada)	**25**	**26**	**27**	**28**	**29**
30	**31** Memorial Day (USA) Spring Bank Holiday (UK)					

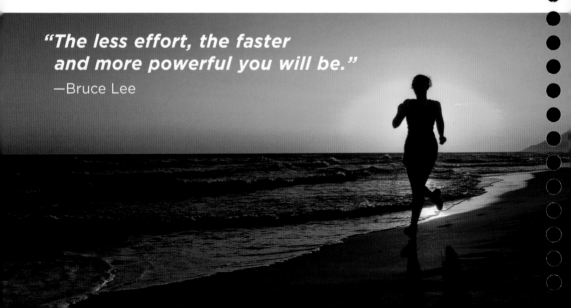

"The less effort, the faster and more powerful you will be."
—Bruce Lee

SHOPPER

Can you resist inhaling the smell of new running shoes before you put them on for their first workout? Their essence hints at victories, long lonely hours on roads at dusk, and a runner being transformed with every quarter mile. They carry your dreams.

Actually, they're just shoes, ugly throw pillows strapped to your feet, and even you won't want to huff them after three months of workouts. Still, it's good to get gushy about running shoes. It cuts through the technical jibber-jabber when shopping for a new pair. Emotions bring wisdom where your feet are concerned. Pains and injuries create a mental diary that you want to take with you to the shoe store.

Also bring along your old pair, no doubt lovely diaries of their own, chronicling your savagery and mad determination. The wear on their outsoles, heel counters, and ankle collars tell an experienced salesperson about the hidden geometry of your body and the idiosyncrasies of your stride and footfall. It will narrow the list of recommended models. Time will be saved. For the moment, do not look at the price, and never, ever consider buying running shoes for their looks.

Shop in the afternoon, if possible (even better, after a run) because your feet swell throughout the day. You want them fully engorged. Have them measured even if you've had them measured 100 times in your adult life. Feet change with age, with your training history, with the weather. Shoes change, too, in design, materials, and quality of manufacture. Measuring your feet is the first date for evaluating a physical connection that is as intimate as sex.

Now plunge into them. Your toes will squabble with each other to issue the first report, but heed your heels instead. Snug is what you want, but what exactly does that mean? Most running shoes have semi-rigid cups that cradle and support your heel while allowing your ankle free travel. They're called heel counters, and contrary to popular belief, they do not provide motion control, though they center your heel for stable landings. Minimalist shoes dispense with them altogether. The choice is up to you. Just make sure your heel doesn't move around too much.

Splay your toes. Arch them. Type out this sentence with them on a make-believe keypad. The toe box on running shoes allows for plenty of wiggle—if the shoes properly fit you. This is because everything forward from your arch changes shape throughout the fluid motion of a stride. Enormous amounts of force and ungainly poundage converge on your feet, ligaments reaching toward the back of your neck. And the only real way to test a running shoe is to . . . run.

Leave the salesclerk a credit card or your child as collateral, and head for the door. Search out as much varied surface as possible. Give yourself plenty of time to get up to a normal tempo, and then fall in love—or try to. If your heart says yes, look at the price tag. Splurge. ∎

Distance carried forward:

26 Monday   116

Where & When: Distance:

Comments:

27 Tuesday   117

Where & When: Distance:

Comments:

28 Wednesday   118

Where & When: Distance:

Comments:

29 Thursday   119

Where & When: Distance:

Comments:

30 Friday   120

Where & When: Distance:

Comments:

121   **Saturday 1**

_____

_____

Where & When: _____ Distance: _____

Comments: _____

_____

122   **Sunday 2**

_____

_____

Where & When: _____ Distance: _____

Comments: _____

_____

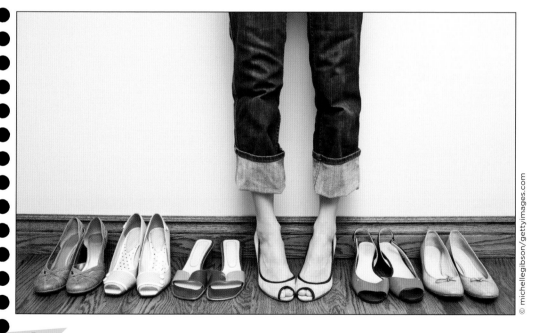

© michellegibson/gettyimages.com

tip: A runner's foot problems often result from daily footwear, not running shoes. Heels, pumps, ballet flats, flip-flops, cowboy boots, and anything with a narrow toe box are primary villains.

Distance this week: _____ Weight: _____

Distance carried forward: _____

3 Monday 123
_____
_____
_____

Where & When: _____ **Distance:** _____
Comments: _____
_____

4 Tuesday 124
_____
_____
_____

Where & When: _____ **Distance:** _____
Comments: _____
_____

5 Wednesday 125
_____
_____
_____

Where & When: _____ **Distance:** _____
Comments: _____
_____

6 Thursday 126
_____
_____
_____

Where & When: _____ **Distance:** _____
Comments: _____
_____

7 Friday 127
_____
_____
_____

Where & When: _____ **Distance:** _____
Comments: _____
_____

May

Saturday 8

Where & When: _____   Distance: _____

Comments: _____

Sunday 9

Where & When: _____   Distance: _____

Comments: _____

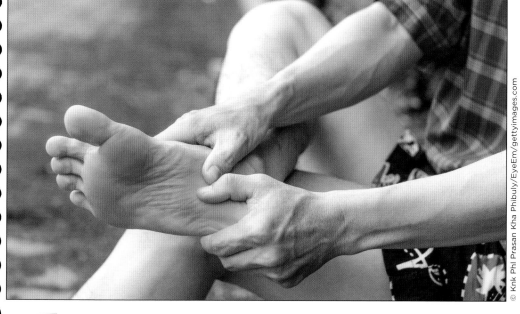

© Knk Phl Prasan Kha Phibuly/EyeEm/gettyimages.com

tip: In treating plantar fasciitis, a seated foot stretch tends to get better results than a standing calf stretch.

Distance this week: _____   **Weight:** _____

Distance carried forward: _____

10 Monday   130

_____
_____
_____

Where & When: _____ **Distance:** _____
Comments: _____
_____

11 Tuesday   131

_____
_____
_____

Where & When: _____ **Distance:** _____
Comments: _____
_____

12 Wednesday   132

_____
_____
_____

Where & When: _____ **Distance:** _____
Comments: _____
_____

13 Thursday   133

_____
_____
_____

Where & When: _____ **Distance:** _____
Comments: _____
_____

14 Friday   134

_____
_____
_____

Where & When: _____ **Distance:** _____
Comments: _____
_____

May

Saturday 15

135

Where & When: _____ Distance: _____

Comments: _____

Sunday 16

136

Where & When: _____ Distance: _____

Comments: _____

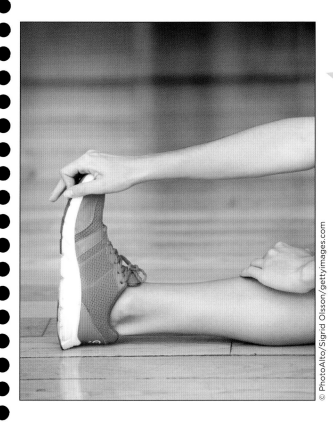

tip: Neither minimalist, barefoot-like shoes, nor maximalist shoes with their fat, thick soles have proven to significantly reduce running injuries.

© PhotoAlto/Sigrid Olsson/gettyimages.com

Distance this week: _____ Weight: _____

Distance carried forward:

17 Monday 137

Where & When: **Distance:**

Comments:

18 Tuesday 138

Where & When: **Distance:**

Comments:

19 Wednesday 139

Where & When: **Distance:**

Comments:

20 Thursday 140

Where & When: **Distance:**

Comments:

21 Friday 141

Where & When: **Distance:**

Comments:

May

Saturday 22

142

Where & When: **Distance:**

Comments:

Sunday 23

143

Where & When: **Distance:**

Comments:

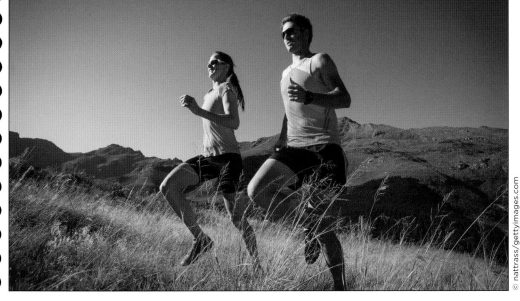

© nattrass/gettyimages.com

tip: Worried about provoking a healed injury again? Shorten your stride and increase your cadence.

Distance this week: **Weight:**

Distance carried forward: _____

24 Monday 144

_____
_____
_____

Where & When: _____ **Distance:** _____
Comments: _____
_____

25 Tuesday 145

_____
_____
_____

Where & When: _____ **Distance:** _____
Comments: _____
_____

26 Wednesday 146

_____
_____
_____

Where & When: _____ **Distance:** _____
Comments: _____
_____

27 Thursday 147

_____
_____
_____

Where & When: _____ **Distance:** _____
Comments: _____
_____

28 Friday 148

_____
_____
_____

Where & When: _____ **Distance:** _____
Comments: _____
_____

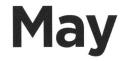

Saturday 29

Where & When: **Distance:**

Comments:

Sunday 30

Where & When: **Distance:**

Comments:

"Recreate your life always, always. Remove the stones, plant rose bushes, make sweets. Begin again."

—Cora Coralina

tip: Experimentation in your training program is an act of humility, an acknowledgment that you can't know how good a runner you are unless you try something different.

Notes:

Distance this week: **Weight:**

June 2021

SUNDAY	MONDAY	TUESDAY	WEDNESDAY	THURSDAY	FRIDAY	SATURDAY
		1	2	3	4	5
6	7 Queen's Birthday (NZ) Western Australia Day Spring Bank Holiday (Ireland)	8	9	10	11	12
13	14 Flag Day (USA) Queen's Birthday (Australia—except QLD, WA)	15	16	17	18	19
20 Father's Day (USA, Canada, Ireland, UK)	21	22	23	24	25	26
27	28	29	30			

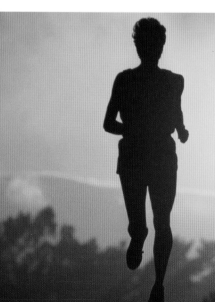

"Keep a little fire burning; however small, however hidden."

—Cormac McCarthy

PRIMA DONNA

Your body doesn't deserve your devotion. Impetuous and demanding, it has made you servile. You indulge it, nurture it, pay for its dinner. In return, you ask for meager but steady progress, a little faster, a little more distance, all prearranged by a honed and accommodating training schedule. You hold up your end of the bargain, yet progress stalls. Your workouts go flatline. Your body balks like a sulking child.

The recommended remedy for training ruts is speedwork. You could also try ice baths, power squats, mud runs, or other tortures to bully your body back in line. Alternatively, you can coax it with compassion and patience, even though it deserves neither. This has given rise to so-called sweet-spot training, in which you cast the bulk of your workouts into a benevolent compromise between distance and intensity. Weekly mileage goes down, and speedwork gets tossed (for the time being). These are replaced by intervals run at 85 to 93 percent of your Functional Threshold Power (FTP). You'll need a fitness tracker or a nerdy coach to get you there.

The pace you're seeking is faster than a tempo run, slower than a threshold sprint. It might take you several weeks to find your magical sweet spot, but it delivers two key benefits. You will continue to build both aerobic capacity and lactate threshold, albeit slowly. Also, it reduces both workout time and agony. In other words, these aren't just maintenance drills. You will get stronger and you will gripe about it less.

Sweet-spot training is particularly useful when you're nervous about an approaching race date and you lag behind the benchmarks of progress you've set. Use the time to tweak or throw out entirely your current workout regimen. Put racing plans on ice. For most runners, this type of training props up a program gone south, allowing time to fix it. While you're tinkering, pay attention to the specific gains you get. Call them Happy Workouts. Performance improves slow and steady, with no tantrums from your peevish body. The chance of injury goes down, too.

Racers must eventually return to speedwork. In fact, any runner striving toward a goal worthy of their workouts will grow impatient with the puny gains from sweet-spot training. You know your body can deliver more and that its insolence will pass. Meanwhile, roll your eyes and hand it your hanky. When its protests subside, only time and dignity will have been lost.

Some runners absolutely love sweet-spot training as a genial road to improvement. The pleasure of working just slightly above your comfort level for extended intervals makes the small gains worth it. You may be astonished at how long you can sustain the effort, how these miles leave you depleted but not flattened. The secret is to guard against complacency. Your sweet spot moves as your performance improves. You must constantly rejigger your workouts.

Also remember that they're not rehab. Injury and illness require a complete overhaul of goals, timetables, and workouts. But when your body is merely petulant and pouting, they can bring back a smile. ■

Distance carried forward:

31 Monday   151

Where & When: Distance:

Comments:

1 Tuesday   152

Where & When: Distance:

Comments:

2 Wednesday   153

Where & When: Distance:

Comments:

3 Thursday   154

Where & When: Distance:

Comments:

4 Friday   155

Where & When: Distance:

Comments:

May/June

Saturday 5

Where & When: **Distance:**

Comments:

Sunday 6

Where & When: **Distance:**

Comments:

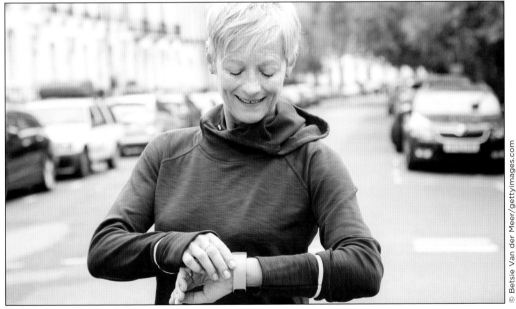

tip: In addition to a reliable heart monitor, better fitness trackers come with a long battery life, GPS, and waterproof design. A sleep-tracking feature is nice as well.

Distance this week: **Weight:**

Distance carried forward:

7 Monday 158

Where & When: Distance:

Comments:

8 Tuesday 159

Where & When: Distance:

Comments:

9 Wednesday 160

Where & When: Distance:

Comments:

10 Thursday 161

Where & When: Distance:

Comments:

11 Friday 162

Where & When: Distance:

Comments:

June

Saturday 12

Where & When: **Distance:**

Comments:

Sunday 13

Where & When: **Distance:**

Comments:

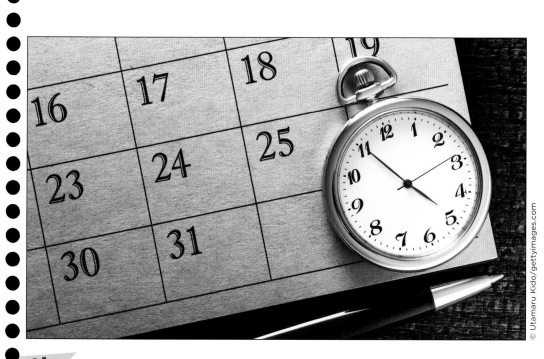

© Utamaru Kido/gettyimages.com

tip: Before committing to any distance race, carefully consider the time you can realistically—week by week—dedicate to training.

Distance this week: **Weight:**

Distance carried forward: _____

14 Monday 165

_____
_____

Where & When: _____ **Distance:** _____
Comments: _____

15 Tuesday 166

_____
_____

Where & When: _____ **Distance:** _____
Comments: _____

16 Wednesday 167

_____
_____

Where & When: _____ **Distance:** _____
Comments: _____

17 Thursday 168

_____
_____

Where & When: _____ **Distance:** _____
Comments: _____

18 Friday 169

_____
_____

Where & When: _____ **Distance:** _____
Comments: _____

June

Saturday 19

Where & When: **Distance:**

Comments:

Sunday 20

Where & When: **Distance:**

Comments:

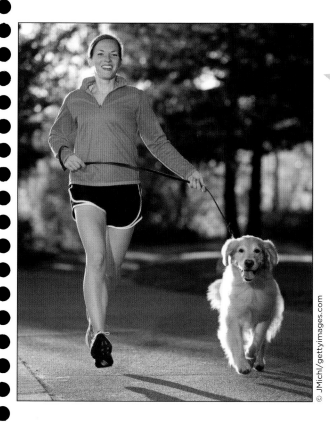

© JMichl/gettyimages.com

tip: If your dog is a workout companion, make sure there are water breaks no more than 30 minutes apart. And don't share your sports drink. It can provoke diarrhea in a pooch.

Distance this week: **Weight:**

Distance carried forward:

21 Monday
172

Where & When: Distance:

Comments:

22 Tuesday
173

Where & When: Distance:

Comments:

23 Wednesday
174

Where & When: Distance:

Comments:

24 Thursday
175

Where & When: Distance:

Comments:

25 Friday
176

Where & When: Distance:

Comments:

June

Saturday 26

Where & When: _____ Distance: _____

Comments: _____

Sunday 27

Where & When: _____ Distance: _____

Comments: _____

"Success is stumbling from failure to failure with no loss of enthusiasm."

—Winston S. Churchill

tip: Mentally respond to setbacks in training with constructive criticism. Make it a habit.

Notes: _____

Distance this week: _____ Weight: _____

July 2021

SUNDAY	MONDAY	TUESDAY	WEDNESDAY	THURSDAY	FRIDAY	SATURDAY
				1 Canada Day	2	3
4 Independence Day (USA)	5	6	7	8	9	10
11	12	13	14	15	16	17
18	19 Eid al-Adha	20	21	22	23	24
25	26	27	28	29	30	31

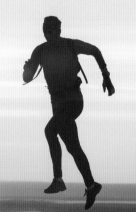

"Heroism is endurance for one moment more."

—George F. Kennon

NUDE

Take it off, all of it. Leave it in the road. However you spend this summer, be a little selfish, a little flagrant. Make it personal. Shed anything that binds you or stands between you and the exuberance of the season.

Start with your calendar. Strip away as many outside commitments as possible so that you can train hard and long. That's what summer is for—unrushed distance, in abrupt morning light or lingering shadows. If you can safely run at night, you will practically hear your thoughts. You will smell at least two things you've never noticed. Share meals and laughs with houseguests this time of year, but make it clear that training time is nonnegotiable. Send flowers or a nice bottle of wine to barbecues you have declined for reasons you have invented.

Now let familiar routines and habits in your training drop away. Run on an empty stomach (it won't kill you). Take an outlandish approach to sun protection with eyewear, hats, wicking shirts, and whatever you drink. Try new routes simply because they're shaded or because they meander around cool bodies of water. Do a long post-workout stretch under the stars. Doff all constraining measures of time, whether in intervals, finishing records, or weeks. The novelties you introduce are less important than what you learn from the stripping away, the bucking of your own inertia, even in little ways.

While you're at it, can you cast off all competitive instincts, especially the ways you compete against yourself? This is harder than it sounds. To a runner, everything is some kind of measured progress, from footfalls to finish lines—or perhaps the days that have passed since you left behind an old way of living. We are always pushing against some transient limit, including the kind with two hairy legs running 100 meters ahead of us. Personal drive is our essence, but it isn't everything. If you can revisit old workouts that were simply satisfying or therapeutic, you may find wellsprings of inspiration when you return to your efficient training mill with its nagging numbers, hopefully after Labor Day.

I see that you haven't fully undressed yet. What else can you shed? Lose the sanctimonious diet for a few weeks (but gorge on summer fruits and vegetables). Most of us don't need rain gear and don't mind rivulets running down our shorts, at least until they chafe. Slip out of your solitude and run with someone who is good company, even if they're a hopeless runner. Or do the opposite: Drop your current partner like sweaty socks into a hamper for languorous workouts in which no voices intrude.

Running is ritual and over time we collect burdensome habits and mindless pieties. You can't know the purity of the runner within until you shed these layers. Summer is the time to do it. ■

Distance carried forward:

28 Monday 179

Where & When: **Distance:**

Comments:

29 Tuesday 180

Where & When: **Distance:**

Comments:

30 Wednesday 181

Where & When: **Distance:**

Comments:

1 Thursday 182

Where & When: **Distance:**

Comments:

2 Friday 183

Where & When: **Distance:**

Comments:

184

Where & When: _____ Distance: _____
Comments: _____

185

Where & When: _____ Distance: _____
Comments: _____

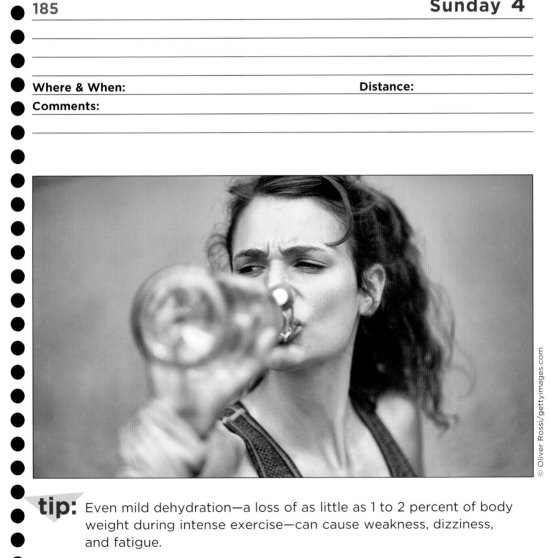

© Oliver Rossi/gettyimages.com

tip: Even mild dehydration—a loss of as little as 1 to 2 percent of body weight during intense exercise—can cause weakness, dizziness, and fatigue.

Distance this week: _____ **Weight:** _____

Distance carried forward:

5 Monday
186

Where & When: Distance:

Comments:

6 Tuesday
187

Where & When: Distance:

Comments:

7 Wednesday
188

Where & When: Distance:

Comments:

8 Thursday
189

Where & When: Distance:

Comments:

9 Friday
190

Where & When: Distance:

Comments:

Saturday 10

191
_____

Where & When: _____ **Distance:** _____

Comments: _____

Sunday 11

192
_____

Where & When: _____ **Distance:** _____

Comments: _____

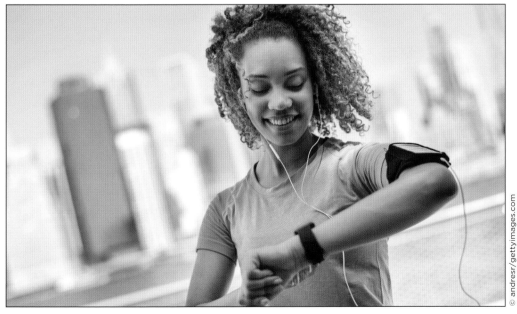

© andresr/gettyimages.com

tip: To get the most from your tracking device, start by identifying your objective. Gathered data will show you what you need to learn or change.

Distance this week: _____ **Weight:** _____

Distance carried forward:

12 Monday 193

Where & When: **Distance:**

Comments:

13 Tuesday 194

Where & When: **Distance:**

Comments:

14 Wednesday 195

Where & When: **Distance:**

Comments:

15 Thursday 196

Where & When: **Distance:**

Comments:

16 Friday 197

Where & When: **Distance:**

Comments:

July

Saturday 17

_____

_____

_____

Where & When: _____ **Distance:** _____

Comments: _____

_____

Sunday 18

_____

_____

_____

Where & When: _____ **Distance:** _____

Comments: _____

_____

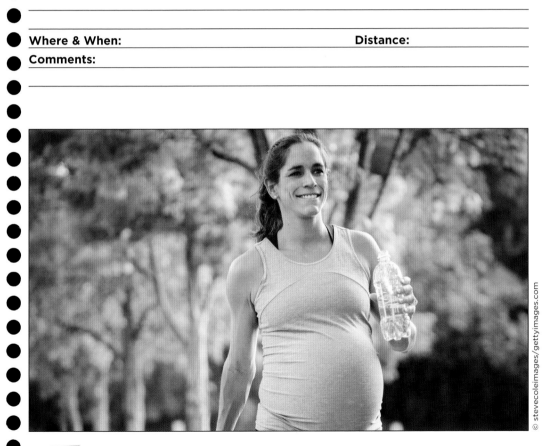

© stevecoleimages/gettyimages.com

tip: Every pregnancy is unique, but many mothers now train into their second trimesters and beyond with healthy pregnancies and few delivery complications. Consult your doctor.

Distance this week: _____ **Weight:** _____

Distance carried forward: _____

19 Monday   200

_____
_____
_____

Where & When: _____ **Distance:** _____
Comments: _____
_____

20 Tuesday   201

_____
_____
_____

Where & When: _____ **Distance:** _____
Comments: _____
_____

21 Wednesday   202

_____
_____
_____

Where & When: _____ **Distance:** _____
Comments: _____
_____

22 Thursday   203

_____
_____
_____

Where & When: _____ **Distance:** _____
Comments: _____
_____

23 Friday   204

_____
_____
_____

Where & When: _____ **Distance:** _____
Comments: _____
_____

205

Where & When: _____ Distance: _____
Comments: _____

206

Where & When: _____ Distance: _____
Comments: _____

"Faith moves mountains, but you have to keep pushing while you are praying."
—Mason Cooley

tip: It's true: Short, highly intense intervals burn more fat than longer, moderate intensity routines.

Notes: _____
_____
_____
_____

Distance this week: _____ **Weight:** _____

August 2021

SUNDAY	MONDAY	TUESDAY	WEDNESDAY	THURSDAY	FRIDAY	SATURDAY
1	2	3	4	5	6	7
	Summer Bank Holiday (Ireland, UK—Scotland, Australia—NSW) Picnic Day (Australia—NT)					
8	9	10	11	12	13	14
15	16	17	18	19	20	21
22	23	24	25	26	27	28
29	30	31				
	Summer Bank Holiday (UK—except Scotland)					

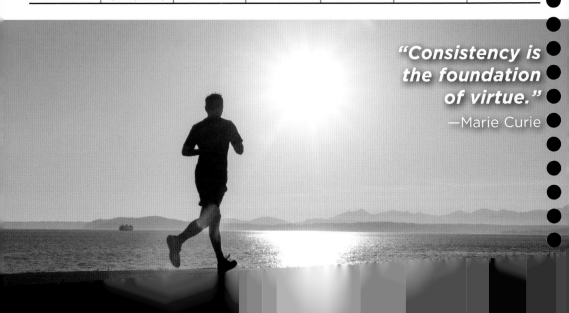

"Consistency is the foundation of virtue."
—Marie Curie

BUTTINSKI

It's a bit of a buzzkill to learn that you don't play as big a role in the whole training thing as you'd like to believe. Most of what makes you the runner you are doesn't happen in the sweat and grind of devoted workouts. The important stuff occurs when you're unconscious, drooling on your pillow.

This is depressing. Recovery begins with the last staggering stride, the first gulp of replenishing liquid. It's where strength building starts. And it's only natural that we'd want to direct and control it in the same ways we lord over our workouts. On this score, we're marginally more useful than hiccups. Yet so keen is the desire to master recovery that both a sports physiology specialty and an industry aspire to aid and enlighten us.

Most of the gear, beverages, supplements, and services for sale are magic beans. They're marketed by entrepreneurs who want your money but don't care enough about whether any of their stuff actually works. Sports recovery is a centuries-old industry of flimflam. The people in lab coats, on the other hand, know a great deal about recovery and continue to reveal more with breathless speed. It's just that they haven't found a way to get you very much involved.

Technically, recovery is the process of restoring your body's homeostasis, a balance of internal conditions, that includes everything from lactate and cortisone levels to hydration, blood flow, and dozens of other things that can be measured. Scientists know what recovery looks like, what it's supposed to look like, and the mess it will make of you if it's out of whack. The great scientific consensus that emerges now advises that to aid in recovery, a runner should drink something when thirsty and get a lot of sleep.

This is not exactly a pioneering pathway in the likes of penicillin or in vitro fertilization, though perhaps that's unfair. Even the ancient Greeks believed in the therapeutic benefits of a post-workout massage. No evidence for that, say modern lab coats, but nor will massage impede the process. Stretching? The jury is out, but if there are benefits, they're minimal. How about compression, either through clothing or with a pulsatile pneumatic device? That would be a no. Cryotherapy (ice baths)? A cold beer is just as effective and generally more pleasant.

The same goes for the nostrums you buy. There's nothing necessarily wrong with the powders and potions that promise quick or triumphant recovery, nor with the many ridiculous things people wear while running. It's just that they don't work—not to any extent that should interest a runner, including elite athletes. When you're hunting for recovery aids and exercises, be aware that many are quite effective at easing pain. Use them. Just remind yourself that ibuprofen and hot tubs do not mend torn muscle tissue or restore cellular glycogen levels. Your body manages these on its own, thank you. While it's busy, it would prefer that you go check your Facebook feed or something. ∎

Distance carried forward: _____

26 Monday   207

_____

_____

_____

Where & When: _____ **Distance:** _____

Comments: _____

_____

27 Tuesday   208

_____

_____

_____

Where & When: _____ **Distance:** _____

Comments: _____

_____

28 Wednesday   209

_____

_____

_____

Where & When: _____ **Distance:** _____

Comments: _____

_____

29 Thursday   210

_____

_____

_____

Where & When: _____ **Distance:** _____

Comments: _____

_____

30 Friday   211

_____

_____

_____

Where & When: _____ **Distance:** _____

Comments: _____

_____

Saturday 31

212

Where & When: Distance:

Comments:

---

213   **Sunday 1**

Where & When: Distance:

Comments:

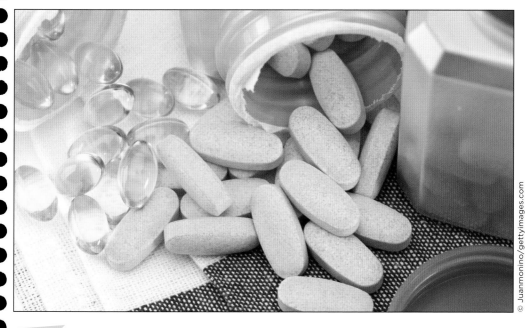

© Juanmonino/gettyimages.com

tip: It's now pretty well established that whatever their upsides, dietary supplements do not extend life.

Distance this week: Weight:

Distance carried forward:

2 Monday 214

Where & When: **Distance:**
Comments:

3 Tuesday 215

Where & When: **Distance:**
Comments:

4 Wednesday 216

Where & When: **Distance:**
Comments:

5 Thursday 217

Where & When: **Distance:**
Comments:

6 Friday 218

Where & When: **Distance:**
Comments:

Saturday 7

219

Where & When: _____ Distance: _____

Comments: _____

220

Sunday 8

Where & When: _____ Distance: _____

Comments: _____

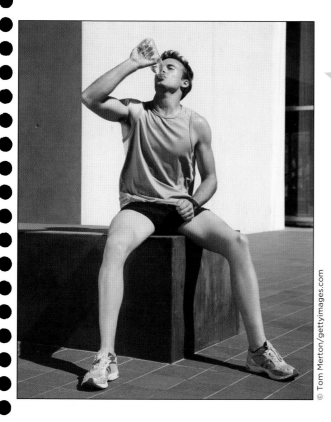

© Tom Merton/gettyimages.com

tip: Unfortunately, the symptoms of overhydration look similar to the symptoms of dehydration—primarily dizziness, confusion, and fatigue.

Distance this week: _____ **Weight:** _____

Distance carried forward:

9 Monday
221

Where & When: Distance:

Comments:

10 Tuesday
222

Where & When: Distance:

Comments:

11 Wednesday
223

Where & When: Distance:

Comments:

12 Thursday
224

Where & When: Distance:

Comments:

13 Friday
225

Where & When: Distance:

Comments:

August

Saturday 14

Where & When: Distance:

Comments:

Sunday 15

Where & When: Distance:

Comments:

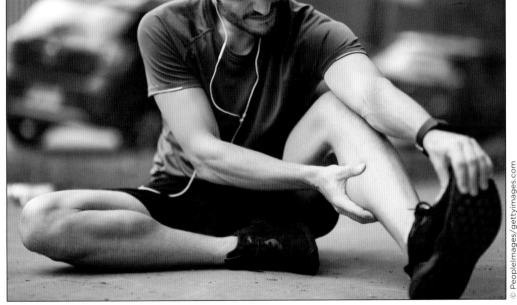

© PeopleImages/gettyimages.com

tip: The vindictive charley horse doesn't cause lasting injury. Dehydration, muscle overuse, nerve irritation, and low levels of certain minerals—like potassium and calcium—can be culprits.

Distance this week: **Weight:**

Distance carried forward: _____

16 Monday   228
_____
_____

Where & When: _____ **Distance:** _____
Comments: _____
_____

17 Tuesday   229
_____
_____

Where & When: _____ **Distance:** _____
Comments: _____
_____

18 Wednesday   230
_____
_____

Where & When: _____ **Distance:** _____
Comments: _____
_____

19 Thursday   231
_____
_____

Where & When: _____ **Distance:** _____
Comments: _____
_____

20 Friday   232
_____
_____

Where & When: _____ **Distance:** _____
Comments: _____
_____

August

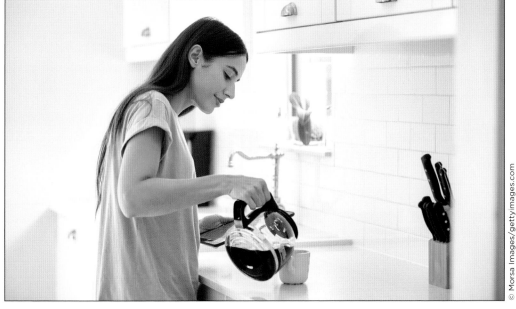

233   **Saturday 21**

Where & When: **Distance:**

Comments:

234   **Sunday 22**

Where & When: **Distance:**

Comments:

© Morsa Images/gettyimages.com

tip: Yup, a big jolt of caffeine one hour before a workout truly boosts performance.

Distance this week: **Weight:**

Distance carried forward:

23 Monday 235

Where & When: Distance:

Comments:

24 Tuesday 236

Where & When: Distance:

Comments:

25 Wednesday 237

Where & When: Distance:

Comments:

26 Thursday 238

Where & When: Distance:

Comments:

27 Friday 239

Where & When: Distance:

Comments:

August

Saturday 28

240

_____

Where & When: _____   Distance: _____
Comments: _____

_____

241

Sunday 29

_____

Where & When: _____   Distance: _____
Comments: _____

_____

"Dwell on the beauty of life. Watch the stars and see yourself running with them."

—Marcus Aurelius

tip: Don't let a single set of data from your fitness tracker distract you from the many other factors that make you a stronger runner.

Notes: _____
_____
_____
_____

Distance this week: _____   **Weight:** _____

September 2021

SUNDAY	MONDAY	TUESDAY	WEDNESDAY	THURSDAY	FRIDAY	SATURDAY
			1	2	3	4
5	6	7	8	9	10	11
Father's Day (Australia, NZ)	Labor Day (USA, Canada)	Rosh Hashanah*	Rosh Hashanah ends			
12	13	14	15	16	17	18
				Yom Kippur*		
19	20	21	22	23	24	25
		U.N. International Day of Peace				
26	27	28	29	30		
	Queen's Birthday (Australia—WA)					

*Begins at sundown the previous day

"If you aren't making some mistakes, you're not taking enough chances."
—John Sculley

TERRAIN

That most sacred place for a runner is surely the shifting contact patch between your shoe sole and the planet hurtling you across the universe. You laugh, yet the aching 3 a.m. walk to the bathroom the morning after a hard run reminds you of your inviolate, sometimes tortured relationship with Earth. For your next workout, perhaps you should reconsider what's underfoot.

Concrete: Hell is paved with concrete. Avoid it here on Earth. Brutally calculable and severe, it shows you at your fastest because it turns you into a human basketball. The energy in every footfall gets bounced right back into the next stride, nothing squandered. The bounce heads upward from feet and ankles through your hips, onto your spine and neck. These frivolous body parts will ache the day following a strenuous workout on concrete, though most evidence suggests you'll suffer little lasting damage.

Asphalt: This is where most of us train. Over time, your feet will become connoisseurs of the stuff. Some surfaces are little more than slightly solidified pea-stone driveways; others are as unyielding as medieval causeways. Asphalt assures consistency in workout results without too much punishment, especially on your Achilles tendon. It also invites complacency and boredom. The heat it radiates in summer months can cook your entire body. Try not to get hit by a car.

Track: The monotony of running on a track is far less than the treadmill and it won't make you feel drunk, as a too-soft conveyer belt will. Tracks are better for short workouts than for distance because running in circles for long periods stresses your iliotibial (IT) band. A good track is an indulgent surface for runners. If you find one, use it often, even if it means trespassing.

Trail: A lot of trail runners have interesting life stories. Who knows why? Trails require puzzle-solving skills, quick improvisation, and sharp but darting focus. How far can you leap? Good trails practically celebrate terrain, the changing seasons throwing wild surprises at you: One workout it's a puddle, the next a pond. If you're new to trails, start slow and maybe get your vision checked beforehand.

Sand and grass: Subsidiaries of trail running, these wicked surfaces beg for dedicated workouts if you can find a sufficient stretch of them. Each uniquely builds speed and balance. Each will try to kill you. The tenuous traction they afford can vary from stride to stride with no visual clues whatsoever. These aren't their only deceptions. They conceal random stones, dog poop, gopher holes, and lawn sprinklers. Outsmarting sand or grass will not bring any runner glory. But the aches in core muscles and proprioceptors the following day point up deficiencies in your regular workouts.

Natural surfaces seduce you to remove your shoes. Go ahead. There's something cosmic about it—your naked vulnerable feet pushing you across the planet, around the sun, through time and space. Your workout somehow seems greater, more connected to everything around you. Just watch out for broken glass. ■

Distance carried forward: _____

30 Monday   242

_____

_____

_____

Where & When: _____ **Distance:** _____

Comments: _____

31 Tuesday   243

_____

_____

_____

Where & When: _____ **Distance:** _____

Comments: _____

1 Wednesday   244

_____

_____

_____

Where & When: _____ **Distance:** _____

Comments: _____

2 Thursday   245

_____

_____

_____

Where & When: _____ **Distance:** _____

Comments: _____

3 Friday   246

_____

_____

_____

Where & When: _____ **Distance:** _____

Comments: _____

Aug/Sept

Saturday 4

Where & When: **Distance:**

Comments:

Sunday 5

Where & When: **Distance:**

Comments:

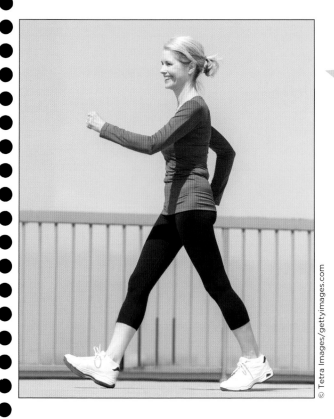

© Tetra Images/gettyimages.com

tip: To clean trail running shoes, sink-wash or spray them with a garden hose, and scrub lightly with a soft-bristled brush dampened with a bit of dish soap. Let them dry by air, not by machine.

Distance this week: **Weight:**

6 Monday

249

Where & When: Distance:

Comments:

7 Tuesday

250

Where & When: Distance:

Comments:

8 Wednesday

251

Where & When: Distance:

Comments:

9 Thursday

252

Where & When: Distance:

Comments:

10 Friday

253

Where & When: Distance:

Comments:

September

Saturday 11

Where & When: _____ Distance: _____

Comments: _____

Sunday 12

Where & When: _____ Distance: _____

Comments: _____

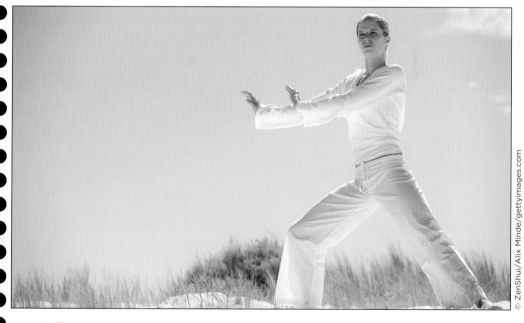

© ZenShui/Alix Minde/gettyimages.com

tip: Trail runners: Tai Chi is excellent for cross-training. It demonstrably improves balance in movement.

Distance this week: _____ Weight: _____

Distance carried forward:

13 Monday 256

Where & When: Distance:

Comments:

14 Tuesday 257

Where & When: Distance:

Comments:

15 Wednesday 258

Where & When: Distance:

Comments:

16 Thursday 259

Where & When: Distance:

Comments:

17 Friday 260

Where & When: Distance:

Comments:

September

Saturday 18

_____

_____

_____

Where & When: _____ **Distance:** _____

Comments: _____

_____

Sunday 19

_____

_____

_____

Where & When: _____ **Distance:** _____

Comments: _____

_____

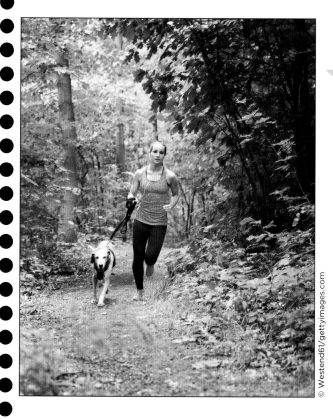

© Westend61/gettyimages.com

tip: Most snake bites result from mutual surprise. For prevention, stay on the trail, keep your dog on a leash, and wear long pants when temperatures rise to 80 degrees or higher in regions where serpents slither.

Distance this week: _____ **Weight:** _____

Distance carried forward: _____

20 Monday 263

_____
_____
_____

Where & When: _____ **Distance:** _____
Comments: _____
_____

21 Tuesday 264

_____
_____
_____

Where & When: _____ **Distance:** _____
Comments: _____
_____

22 Wednesday 265

_____
_____
_____

Where & When: _____ **Distance:** _____
Comments: _____
_____

23 Thursday 266

_____
_____
_____

Where & When: _____ **Distance:** _____
Comments: _____
_____

24 Friday 267

_____
_____
_____

Where & When: _____ **Distance:** _____
Comments: _____
_____

September

Saturday 25

Where & When: _____ Distance: _____

Comments: _____

Sunday 26

Where & When: _____ Distance: _____

Comments: _____

"To dare is to lose one's footing momentarily. To not dare is to lose oneself."

—Søren Kierkegaard

tip: There's at least some evidence that compression garments—which squeeze your muscles like sausage casings—speed workout recovery. They do not demonstrably improve performance.

Notes: _____

Distance this week: _____ Weight: _____

October 2021

SUNDAY	MONDAY	TUESDAY	WEDNESDAY	THURSDAY	FRIDAY	SATURDAY
					1	2
3	4 Labour Day (Australia—ACT, SA, NSW) Queen's Birthday (Australia—QLD)	5	6	7	8	9
10	11 Columbus Day (USA) Thanksgiving (Canada)	12	13	14	15	16
17	18	19	20	21	22	23
24 United Nations Day **31** Halloween	25 Labour Day (NZ) Bank Holiday (Ireland)	26	27	28	29	30

"What we change inwardly will change outer reality."
—Plutarch

BOMB

Pray for ruin. When you fail at a goal, the last thing you want is ambiguity, dusting yourself off in the aftermath with shrugging acceptance. An uncertain flop means that somewhere in your preparations, you duped yourself. It's better to implode with resounding disgrace, even tears, because crushing defeat is both a map and a compass. It points the way to redemption.

Once you've bushwhacked through the excuses and legitimate circumstances that produced your disaster, you'll blame yourself. The usual sins are wavering determination, bluster, or stupidity. To be sure, truth lurks in these recriminations, but blame is a dead end. It certainly won't make you a better runner. Failure usually shows up early in a training program. Runners ignore the signs because of the time they've already invested, the personal stake from ego and desire. A performance breakthrough will surely arrive in a matter of workouts. What does it say about personal character to dump a dream like a child frustrated with an unyielding toy?

Remind yourself that quitting and failing are two different things, each a blow to the ego. So choose your punishment but remember that quitting doesn't make you a chump. It's a valid solution to a training problem. Winners are merely runners who know when to stop.

Next, rewrite the story of your failure. This may sound like a politician's dodge, but it's actually a way to reveal an achievable goal. Training time wasted on a bum idea is an investment in disguise. Consider it a gift of enlightenment from the runner you used to be. You will reasonably want to review the mistakes that led to your fiasco—as well you should—but dwelling on them spins a distorted narrative. No doubt a number of factors came into play. Just as important are the things that went right. These get forgotten in the pity and woe that well up from defeat.

Now that you're on your feet again, reflect on your comebacks, even those that had nothing to do with running. Humiliation comes in many party sizes, from awkward first dates to an unexpected job loss. Comebacks sometimes bring both triumph and vindication. Children may hose you in video games, but see what happens when you sit the same kids down to a poker table or a Scrabble board. With the right competition, you can take anyone's lunch money.

In other words, defeat is relative and usually temporary. This should give you hope, which is a crucial part of redemption. We commonly speak of optimism as a disposition, a gift to the naive or a smile from the heavens. In fact, it's a practice. You have to work at it (some of us harder than others). One proven strategy is to train with other runners after a major setback. No one really knows why. Perhaps the empathy that comes from shared struggle puts a defeat into manageable perspective. It inspires a faith that you can overcome the failure. Then again, training itself should give you reason to believe. ■

Distance carried forward: _____

27 Monday   270
_____
_____
_____

Where & When: _____ **Distance:** _____
Comments: _____
_____

28 Tuesday   271
_____
_____
_____

Where & When: _____ **Distance:** _____
Comments: _____
_____

29 Wednesday   272
_____
_____
_____

Where & When: _____ **Distance:** _____
Comments: _____
_____

30 Thursday   273
_____
_____
_____

Where & When: _____ **Distance:** _____
Comments: _____
_____

1 Friday   274
_____
_____
_____

Where & When: _____ **Distance:** _____
Comments: _____
_____

275   **Saturday 2**

Where & When: **Distance:**

Comments:

276   **Sunday 3**

Where & When: **Distance:**

Comments:

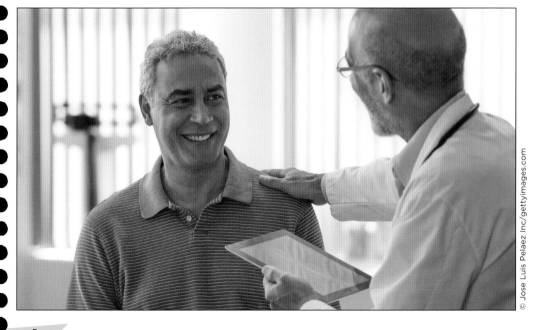

© Jose Luis Pelaez Inc/gettyimages.com

tip: If you're over 50 and returning to running after more than seven years of absence, first have a chat with your doctor about your family medical history and your current health.

Distance this week: **Weight:**

Distance carried forward: _____

4 Monday   277
_____
_____
_____

Where & When: _____ **Distance:** _____
Comments: _____
_____

5 Tuesday   278
_____
_____
_____

Where & When: _____ **Distance:** _____
Comments: _____
_____

6 Wednesday   279
_____
_____
_____

Where & When: _____ **Distance:** _____
Comments: _____
_____

7 Thursday   280
_____
_____
_____

Where & When: _____ **Distance:** _____
Comments: _____
_____

8 Friday   281
_____
_____
_____

Where & When: _____ **Distance:** _____
Comments: _____
_____

October

Saturday 9

_____

_____

_____

Where & When: _____ **Distance:** _____

Comments: _____

_____

Sunday 10

_____

_____

_____

Where & When: _____ **Distance:** _____

Comments: _____

_____

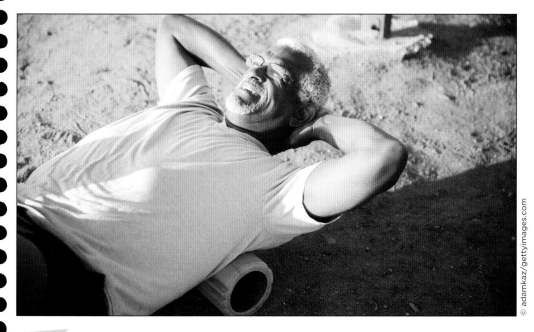

© adamkaz/gettyimages.com

tip: The aging runner's secret recovery weapon? A foam roller.

Distance this week: _____ **Weight:** _____

Distance carried forward:

11 Monday
284

Where & When: **Distance:**

Comments:

12 Tuesday
285

Where & When: **Distance:**

Comments:

13 Wednesday
286

Where & When: **Distance:**

Comments:

14 Thursday
287

Where & When: **Distance:**

Comments:

15 Friday
288

Where & When: **Distance:**

Comments:

October

Saturday 16

_____
_____
_____

Where & When: _____ **Distance:** _____
Comments: _____

Sunday 17

_____
_____
_____

Where & When: _____ **Distance:** _____
Comments: _____

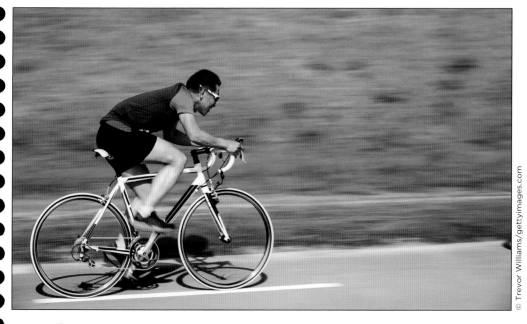

© Trevor Williams/gettyimages.com

tip: Sure, cycling is great for cross training because it's a low-impact exercise. It also lets you work neglected leg muscles without making them support your full body weight.

Distance this week: _____ **Weight:** _____

18 Monday 291

Where & When: Distance:

Comments:

19 Tuesday 292

Where & When: Distance:

Comments:

20 Wednesday 293

Where & When: Distance:

Comments:

21 Thursday 294

Where & When: Distance:

Comments:

22 Friday 295

Where & When: Distance:

Comments:

October

296

_____
_____
_____

Where & When: _____   **Distance:** _____
Comments: _____

297

Sunday 24

_____
_____
_____

Where & When: _____   **Distance:** _____
Comments: _____

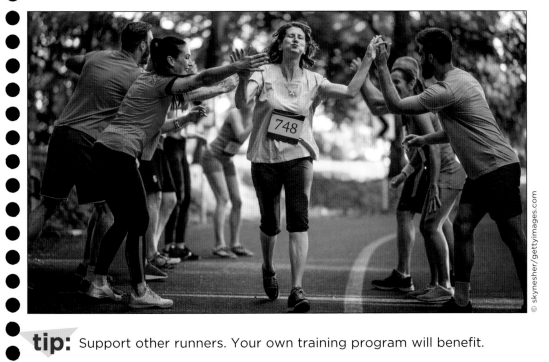

© skynesher/gettyimages.com

tip: Support other runners. Your own training program will benefit.

Distance this week: _____   **Weight:** _____

Distance carried forward:

25 Monday 298

Where & When: Distance:

Comments:

26 Tuesday 299

Where & When: Distance:

Comments:

27 Wednesday 300

Where & When: Distance:

Comments:

28 Thursday 301

Where & When: Distance:

Comments:

29 Friday 302

Where & When: Distance:

Comments:

October

Where & When: _____ Distance: _____

Comments: _____

Where & When: _____ Distance: _____

Comments: _____

*"A river cuts through rock, not because of its power,
but because of its persistence."*
—James N. Watkins

tip: Running before breakfast may guard against weight gain since your body burns from fat stores when carbs aren't available.

Notes: _____

Distance this week: _____ Weight: _____

November 2021

SUNDAY	MONDAY	TUESDAY	WEDNESDAY	THURSDAY	FRIDAY	SATURDAY
	1	2	3	4	5	6
		Election Day (USA)				
7	8	9	10	11	12	13
				Veterans' Day (USA) Remembrance Day (Canada, Ireland, UK)		
14	15	16	17	18	19	20
21	22	23	24	25	26	27
				Thanksgiving (USA)		
28	29	30				
	Hanukkah*	St. Andrew's Day (UK)				

*Begins at sundown the previous day

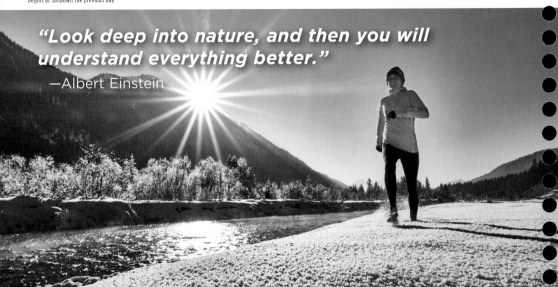

"Look deep into nature, and then you will understand everything better."
—Albert Einstein

MOONSHINE

You're not alone in your dread of winter training. Everyone hates it, except the obnoxious runners who also experience euphoria by running up and down stadium steps until they vomit. No matter where you live, the season presents less pain and danger than summer months. It's mostly a psychological aversion. The ice and slop, the leaflessness and narrow spectrum of reds and grays hardly invite an exuberant, driving workout. Diminished light is the culprit. This year try to make the darkness work for you.

You can winterize your training by adapting it in the months when you're still wearing sandals and eating watermelon. Winter is the time for focused, solemn attention to rehab and strength training. The payoff will burst upon you with the welcome surprise of spring lilacs when you return to normal extended workouts. Variety and specificity are key—exercises and drills you can do indoors and outdoors, at the gym and under your own roof. Cheat the night with squats, planks, back extensions, lunges, and leg lifts. Indulge long stretching sessions with all the lights turned off.

Does this sound as if you're just piddling around? You have every reason to assume so. Any kind of cross-training is as barren to a runner's imagination as a fallow cornfield in November, especially strength building and rehab. You will pursue them as duty, not passion. So if you want them to make you a better runner, you have to set metrics—targets and benchmarks. Make these specific.

Make them progressive. Crowd them together on your calendar. And ensure there are consequences if you fail to meet them (no leftover pecan pie for you, Slacker).

Then there's the treadmill. No runner is neutral about these medieval torture contraptions. Some runners convert to them and never return to pavement. Many don't use them at all. Whatever your opinion, be open to changing it— as your goals and abilities evolve, and even from year to year. At the very least, they're a diversion, and you can blast your music. They are dutiful for sustaining, even advancing, aerobic fitness. They're useful for keeping you in a groove—i.e., pacing. You can work them hard well after twilight, even occasionally in the middle of the night (recommended). And contrary to how they sometimes make you feel, they're not really mocking your running goals, your abilities, or the trajectory of your career and, well, your life.

Conventional wisdom maintains that with limited daylight hours, winter workouts should focus on speedwork. Yes, but wet and icy conditions should likewise make you mindful of bleeding knees and pulled groin muscles. Meanwhile, don't count out competition. November was invented for 5K and 10K races (don't be snobby about your town's annual turkey trot). For that matter, consider springing for an airplane ticket to a race where it's pleasant. And to savor winter light in its sublime, stingy sanctity, at least once in your life, begin your workout 15 minutes before dawn. ■

1 Monday 305

Where & When: Distance:

Comments:

2 Tuesday 306

Where & When: Distance:

Comments:

3 Wednesday 307

Where & When: Distance:

Comments:

4 Thursday 308

Where & When: Distance:

Comments:

5 Friday 309

Where & When: Distance:

Comments:

November

Saturday 6

Where & When: _____ Distance: _____

Comments: _____

Sunday 7

Where & When: _____ Distance: _____

Comments: _____

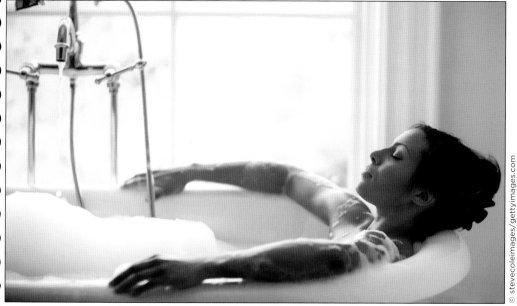

© stevecoleimages/gettyimages.com

tip: When traveling to a warm- or hot-weather race with no time to acclimate, two or three long hot-water baths in the days leading up to the event can help.

Distance this week: _____ Weight: _____

Distance carried forward:

8 Monday 312

Where & When: Distance:
Comments:

9 Tuesday 313

Where & When: Distance:
Comments:

10 Wednesday 314

Where & When: Distance:
Comments:

11 Thursday 315

Where & When: Distance:
Comments:

12 Friday 316

Where & When: Distance:
Comments:

November

317

Where & When: _____ Distance: _____

Comments: _____

318

Where & When: _____ Distance: _____

Comments: _____

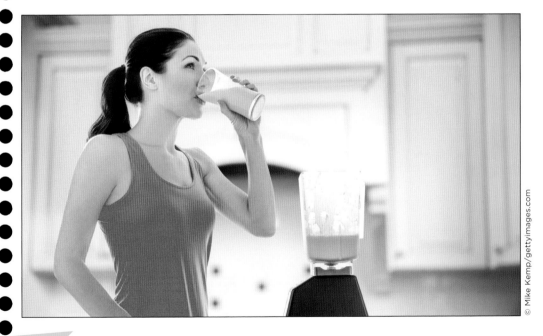

© Mike Kemp/gettyimages.com

tip: Smoothies may seem like excellent pre-workout fuel. But many are loaded with sugar, which your body burns through quickly and can lead to an energy crash. Same with many energy drinks.

Distance this week: _____ Weight: _____

15 Monday

Where & When: **Distance:**

Comments:

16 Tuesday

Where & When: **Distance:**

Comments:

17 Wednesday

Where & When: **Distance:**

Comments:

18 Thursday

Where & When: **Distance:**

Comments:

19 Friday

Where & When: **Distance:**

Comments:

November

324

Where & When: _____ Distance: _____

Comments: _____

325

Where & When: _____ Distance: _____

Comments: _____

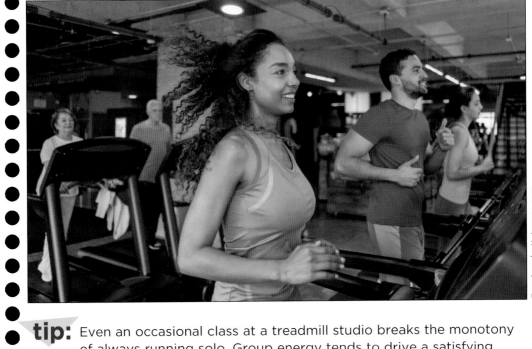

© andresr/gettyimages.com

tip: Even an occasional class at a treadmill studio breaks the monotony of always running solo. Group energy tends to drive a satisfying workout.

Distance this week: _____ Weight: _____

Distance carried forward: _____

22 Monday 326

_____
_____
_____

Where & When: _____ **Distance:** _____
Comments: _____
_____

23 Tuesday 327

_____
_____
_____

Where & When: _____ **Distance:** _____
Comments: _____
_____

24 Wednesday 328

_____
_____
_____

Where & When: _____ **Distance:** _____
Comments: _____
_____

25 Thursday 329

_____
_____
_____

Where & When: _____ **Distance:** _____
Comments: _____
_____

26 Friday 330

_____
_____
_____

Where & When: _____ **Distance:** _____
Comments: _____
_____

November

331

Where & When: _____ Distance: _____

Comments: _____

332   Sunday 28

Where & When: _____ Distance: _____

Comments: _____

"Small change, small wonders—these are the currency of my endurance and ultimately of my life."
—Barbara Kingsolver

tip: Running builds bone strength by generating sudden, sharp forces that bow the affected bones. This kick-starts processes that increase the number of bone cells. See, the training effect goes right to your marrow.

Notes: _____

Distance this week: _____ Weight: _____

December 2021

SUNDAY	MONDAY	TUESDAY	WEDNESDAY	THURSDAY	FRIDAY	SATURDAY
			1	2	3	4
5	6	7	8	9	10	11
	Hanukkah ends				Human Rights Day	
12	13	14	15	16	17	18
19	20	21	22	23	24 Christmas Eve	25 Christmas Day
26 Kwanzaa begins (USA) Boxing Day (Canada, NZ, UK, Australia—except SA) St. Stephen's Day (Ireland)	27 Christmas Day (observed) (NZ, UK, Australia)	28 Boxing Day (observed) (NZ, UK, Australia— except SA) Proclamation Day (observed) (Australia—SA)	29	30	31	

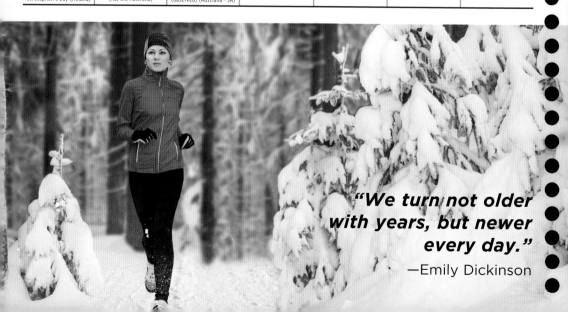

"We turn not older with years, but newer every day."

—Emily Dickinson

SCROOGE

Get to know your ghosts. They hang out with the medals and trophies collecting dust in some back room with all your other personal junk. Or they're wearing that slinky knit number buried in your closet that you worked so hard to fit into, the occasions for it now just mixed memories. Your ghosts are the various runners you used to be, and as your years accrue, their number multiplies.

They will remind you that life comes with an expiration date. Also, you're only as good as your last achievement. Ghosts make a good sounding board when you're planning next year's training. Your abilities change over the years, and so do your passions, judgments, the nature of risks you're willing to take, and the ways you find satisfaction. Your body changes, too. All of these transmogrifications should inform the goals you set. You "contain multitudes," said Walt Whitman. Prove it.

Life events completely unrelated to running change your relationship to it over the years. Try this: Identify a success from your past that still brings a smile to your face. Now recall as much as you can about the context of your life at the time you were training for it—the jeans you wore and the shows you watched, relationships that were particularly close, or the things that kept you up at night. Evoke as much detail as you can. How did training fit in with everything else that was going on?

There are runners who know the very moment when they have set their last personal record—end of running, full stop—no need to justify it to anyone. All athletes want to make a dignified exit, and they want to make the decision themselves. There are also runners who cannot not train. A generation of crazy coots would kindly like you to get out of the way on running trails and high-school tracks. They may not make the prettiest of sights, but you can bet that motivation for runners in their 80s and 90s goes deep, mysteriously deep. No one runs simply out of habit.

When you recognize that you've achieved your last personal record or that you no longer care about wearing slinky knit things, confront the moment. Does training describe something you do or someone you are? Your answer better be good, because it often signals a change in life direction that becomes apparent only years after it has been made. Most of us evolve our running goals to our age and abilities. But there comes a point when the goals no longer motivate, the training fails to reward. It's okay to be a little frightened at the recognition, to be deeply disappointed, and maybe a little angry. But it shouldn't take any runner by surprise.

How you react to the moment says worlds about your essential character. Barring a physical calamity, you won't need to respond right away. But the question hangs over us all. In small ways, it should make you cherish every workout, every opportunity to run. ■

Distance carried forward:

29 Monday   333

Where & When: Distance:

Comments:

30 Tuesday   334

Where & When: Distance:

Comments:

1 Wednesday   335

Where & When: Distance:

Comments:

2 Thursday   336

Where & When: Distance:

Comments:

3 Friday   337

Where & When: Distance:

Comments:

Saturday 4

338

Where & When: Distance:

Comments:

Sunday 5

339

Where & When: Distance:

Comments:

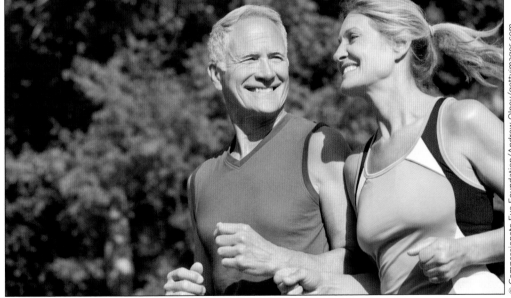

© Compassionate Eye Foundation/Andrew Olney/gettyimages.com

tip: Evidence suggests that older runners benefit from interval training in overall fitness even more than young athletes.

Distance this week: Weight:

Distance carried forward: _____

6 Monday

340

_____
_____

Where & When: **Distance:**
Comments:
_____

7 Tuesday

341

_____
_____

Where & When: **Distance:**
Comments:
_____

8 Wednesday

342

_____
_____

Where & When: **Distance:**
Comments:
_____

9 Thursday

343

_____
_____

Where & When: **Distance:**
Comments:
_____

10 Friday

344

_____
_____

Where & When: **Distance:**
Comments:
_____

December

345   Saturday 11

Where & When: Distance:

Comments:

346   Sunday 12

Where & When: Distance:

Comments:

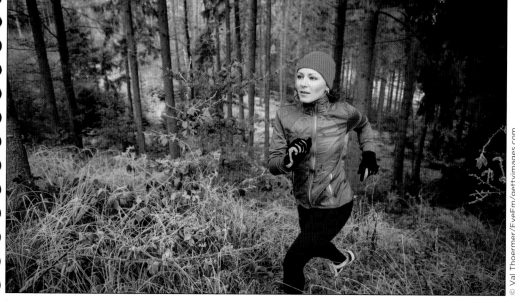

© Val Thoermer/EyeEm/gettyimages.com

tip: Your body eventually adapts to cold-weather workouts. As you wait for it to change, get used to wearing multiple layers.

Distance this week: Weight:

13 Monday   347

Where & When: Distance:
Comments:

14 Tuesday   348

Where & When: Distance:
Comments:

15 Wednesday   349

Where & When: Distance:
Comments:

16 Thursday   350

Where & When: Distance:
Comments:

17 Friday   351

Where & When: Distance:
Comments:

December

Saturday 18

Where & When: Distance:

Comments:

Sunday 19

Where & When: Distance:

Comments:

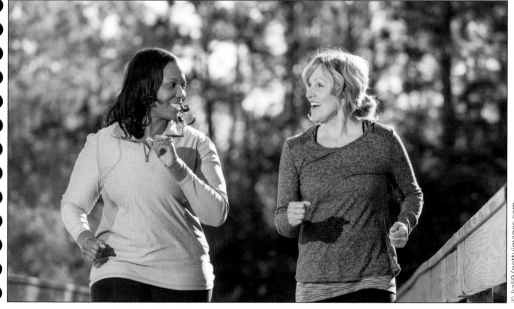

© kali9/gettyimages.com

tip: Physical fitness in middle age is tied to a lower risk of later-life depression and death from cardiovascular disease.

Distance this week: Weight:

Distance carried forward:

20 Monday 354

Where & When: Distance:

Comments:

21 Tuesday 355

Where & When: Distance:

Comments:

22 Wednesday 356

Where & When: Distance:

Comments:

23 Thursday 357

Where & When: Distance:

Comments:

24 Friday 358

Where & When: Distance:

Comments:

December

Saturday 25

Where & When: Distance:
Comments:

Sunday 26

Where & When: Distance:
Comments:

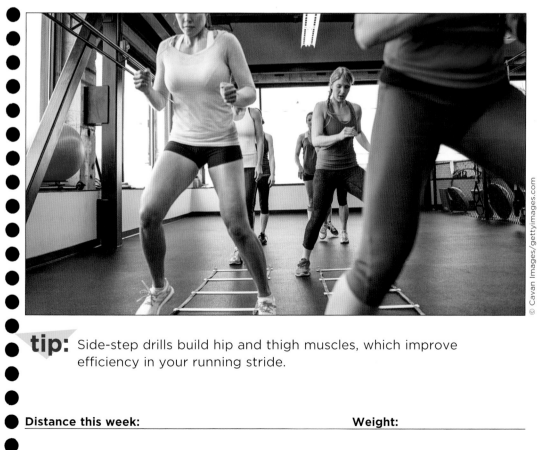

© Cavan Images./gettyimages.com

tip: Side-step drills build hip and thigh muscles, which improve efficiency in your running stride.

Distance this week: **Weight:**

Distance carried forward: _____

27 Monday   361
_____

_____

_____

Where & When: _____ **Distance:** _____
Comments: _____

_____

28 Tuesday   362
_____

_____

_____

Where & When: _____ **Distance:** _____
Comments: _____

_____

29 Wednesday   363
_____

_____

_____

Where & When: _____ **Distance:** _____
Comments: _____

_____

30 Thursday   364
_____

_____

_____

Where & When: _____ **Distance:** _____
Comments: _____

_____

31 Friday   365
_____

_____

_____

Where & When: _____ **Distance:** _____
Comments: _____

Dec/Jan 2022

Saturday 1

Where & When: _____ Distance: _____

Comments: _____

Sunday 2

Where & When: _____ Distance: _____

Comments: _____

"Only those who risk going too far can possibly find out how far one can go."

—T.S. Eliot

tip: Runners over 50 benefit greatly from weight training, which rebuilds naturally declining muscle mass.

Notes: _____

Distance this week: _____ Weight: _____

Twelve Months of Running

Dec. 28	Jan. 4	Jan. 11	Jan. 18	Jan. 25	Feb. 1	Feb. 8	Feb. 15	Feb. 22	March 1	March 8	March 15	March 22

To create a cumulative bar graph of weekly mileage,
apply an appropriate scale at the left-hand margin.
Then fill in the bar for each week of running.

March 29	Apr. 5	Apr. 12	Apr. 19	Apr. 26	May 3	May 10	May 17	May 24	May 31	June 7	June 14	June 21

To create a cumulative bar graph of weekly mileage,
apply an appropriate scale at the left-hand margin.
Then fill in the bar for each week of running.

June 28	July 5	July 12	July 19	July 26	Aug. 2	Aug. 9	Aug. 16	Aug. 23	Aug. 30	Sept. 6	Sept. 13	Sept. 20

To create a cumulative bar graph of weekly mileage,
apply an appropriate scale at the left-hand margin.
Then fill in the bar for each week of running.

Sept. 27	Oct. 4	Oct. 11	Oct. 18	Oct. 25	Nov. 1	Nov. 8	Nov. 15	Nov. 22	Nov. 29	Dec. 6	Dec. 13	Dec. 20	Dec. 27

A Record of Races

Date	Place	Distance	Time	Pace	Comments & Excuses

A Record of Races

Date	Place	Distance	Time	Pace	Comments & Excuses

RACING

Pace is crucial. And you won't magically find it on race day. If you've resisted using a stopwatch or a heart monitor in your workouts, training for a 10K race is the perfect opportunity to abandon those prejudices.

Divide the race into three equal segments and start slower than you want. Don't reach your race pace until the second segment. Push on the third. But your times between these three segments shouldn't vary by more than 10 percent.

10K

Warm up? Yes, even a slow half-mile run before the race is likely to improve your performance, not fatigue you. Remember that a 10K event is too short to grant you a sufficient warm-up during the race.

Half Marathon

If you're running a half-marathon as preparation for a marathon, cut your weekly long run to no more than 12 miles and raise the pace.

Every week should include three types of workouts: speed drills, tempo runs, and your long run. Speed drills make you faster. Tempo runs raise your lactate threshold, which will help you maintain a racing pace in the second half of the event. And your weekly long run increases endurance. Toss in some cross training when time allows.

Don't be shaken by early mistakes. If you go out too fast, for example, simply dial back as soon as you recognize your error. It's a long race and there's plenty of time to recover from just about any kind of blunder.

Marathon

No one masters the marathon. Anything can happen on its long tortuous course, which is why it is such a seductive and exciting event. It's in your interest to arrive at the starting line with this humility.

Seek support. Train with a partner or a running group. Get your loved ones to cheer you on at the race. Raise money for a cause. The road to the marathon can be long and lonely. Let others help you get there.

Believe it or not, it's better to undertrain than to overtrain. What you haven't developed by race day can sometimes be overcome with adrenalin and desire. For an overtrained runner, the race is over before it starts.

Get used to crowding. In open water where visibility is often poor, contact with other swimmers is inevitable. On bicycles it can be dangerous. Patience pays. Fighting through a pack of competitors wastes energy and can throw your race into jeopardy. Relax. Your opportunity to pass will come.

Triathlon

Rehearse transitions. Without specific training, it takes bicycling legs longer to reach their running stride than many athletes realize. Pulling dry socks onto wet feet can be an ordeal. Fussing with uncooperative equipment squanders time.

Your weakest event deserves the greatest amount of training effort. Sorry, it's true. Most triathletes use their best event to make up time. The better strategy is not to lose time in your weak event.

JANUARY 2022

_____
_____
_____
_____
_____

FEBRUARY 2022

_____
_____
_____
_____
_____

MARCH 2022

_____
_____
_____
_____
_____

APRIL 2022

_____
_____
_____
_____
_____

MAY 2022

_____
_____
_____
_____
_____

JUNE 2022

_____
_____
_____
_____
_____

JULY 2022

_____
_____
_____
_____
_____

AUGUST 2022

_____
_____
_____
_____
_____

SEPTEMBER 2022

_____
_____
_____
_____
_____

OCTOBER 2022

_____
_____
_____
_____
_____

NOVEMBER 2022

_____
_____
_____
_____
_____

DECEMBER 2022

_____
_____
_____
_____
_____